# Indian Head Massage

# Indian Head Massage

## DISCOVER THE POWER OF TOUCH

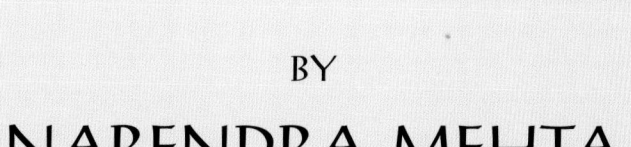

BY

# NARENDRA MEHTA

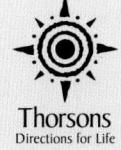

Thorsons
Directions for Life

Thorsons
An Imprint of HarperCollins*Publishers*
77–85 Fulham Palace Road,
Hammersmith, London W6 8JB

The Thorsons website address is:
www.thorsons.com

Published by Thorsons 1999
This edition 2000

10

A catalogue record for this book
is available from the British Library

ISBN 13 978–0–7225–3940–8
ISBN 10 0–7225–3940–1
Photography by Simon McComb
Additional photography by Tony Stone Images
Medical illustration by Peter Cox Associates
Text illustration by Jane Spencer

Printed and bound in China by Imago

**Disclaimer**

This book is intended for people to learn Indian head massage for personal use by following the instructions given herein. Indian head massage is very easy to use, but it must be treated with respect and instructions followed carefully, if they are to be safe and effective. Indian head massage should only be used on your friends and colleagues who are not currently suffering from any chronic or acute problems, such as whiplash injuries, migraine, epilepsy, psoriasis or eczema. If you have an acute or chronic disease or physical pain, then please seek medical attention from a professional therapist or doctor. Although the techniques described here are effective in most cases, they should not be used for medical diagnoses. Indian head massage is a very safe and beneficial therapy, but it is not intended to be a substitute for medical care and treatment.

Please remember that this guide does not in any way replace hands-on professional training. In order to practice professionally, you must first complete an approved training course.

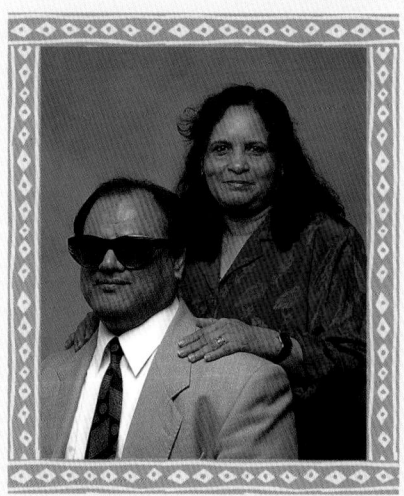

This book is dedicated to my wife, Kundan Mehta, for
her continuous love, support and encouragement.

# Acknowledgements

There are many people to whom I owe a lot, but they are too numerous to name here. I will limit myself to those who have directly contributed to this book in particular and to my career and life in general.

I would like to thank all my students for their encouragement to write this book; my friend Charlotte Wayne for her continuous help and support; Keith Heatherly for assisting me in teaching and researching the subject; Sally McNally and Anita Woodward for their work in promoting the therapy in different parts of the country; Norman MacCallum and Natasha Martyn-Johns for their research and assistance in editing this book; Belinda Budge, Nicky Vimpany and others at Thorsons; and last but not least, grateful thanks to my parents Kantilal and Subhadra Mehta, my uncle and aunt in London, Gopaldas and Bhanuben Desai and my uncle and aunt in Bombay, Ramaniklal and Santaben Mehta all of whom have been a constant source of encouragement and support throughout my career.

# Author's Note

I have been totally blind from the age of one. From my clients' point of view, my blindness is no drawback. Once you're seated in my chair, my fingers do all the seeing I require. I graduated in political science from Bombay University and have been practising bodywork for the last 25 years. I am qualified in body massage, reflexology, touch for health and oesteopathy. I now practise at two London clinics in addition to my own London Centre of Indian Champissage at the Eastern Health and Beauty Centre, 136 Holloway Rd, London, N7 8DD, telephone: 0171 609 3590, fax: 0171 607 4228.

I have described in this book a few simple and effective techniques for you to try out to see the efficacy of this wonderful therapy. I am sure you will be very happy with the result. The beauty of this therapy is that it can be used anywhere all you need is a comfortable chair, and a pair of warm, healing hands. I believe everyone has healing hands all you need is to follow the instructions carefully and allow the healing to flow. You will be pleasantly surprised by the result. Always start with light pressure, gradually increasing it as the recipient feels comfortable. Please do ask the recipient to let you know if and when your pressure is too heavy or too light, or if they are feeling uncomfortable in any way. Indian head massage is easy to give and a pleasure to receive. Have fun!

# FOREWORD

I feel proud to be able to bring this ancient therapy of Indian head massage to the West, and I feel sure that it will make a great contribution to the well-being of humankind. Today, at the London Centre of Indian Champissage, we provide treatments and educational training courses that help spread the therapy further afield. Since I have developed the techniques of Indian head massage to include subtle energy massage, and created the new therapy I call Champissage, its popularity has increased and more and more people are discovering that this therapy provides help for and relief from an ever-increasing range of symptoms.

I have already travelled through several European countries to teach Champissage, including Cyprus, Greece, Spain and Sweden and it has taken off in these countries with rapid success. In the near future, I plan to travel worldwide, especially to America and Canada, to promote this wonderful therapy further.

As a principle of the London Centre of Indian Champissage I am always interested to hear of any scientific research into the effects of this therapy on problems such as drug addiction, depression, insomnia, headaches and migraines, and stress, which are prevalent in our modern society.

Indian Champissage is the therapy of the future.

# CONTENTS

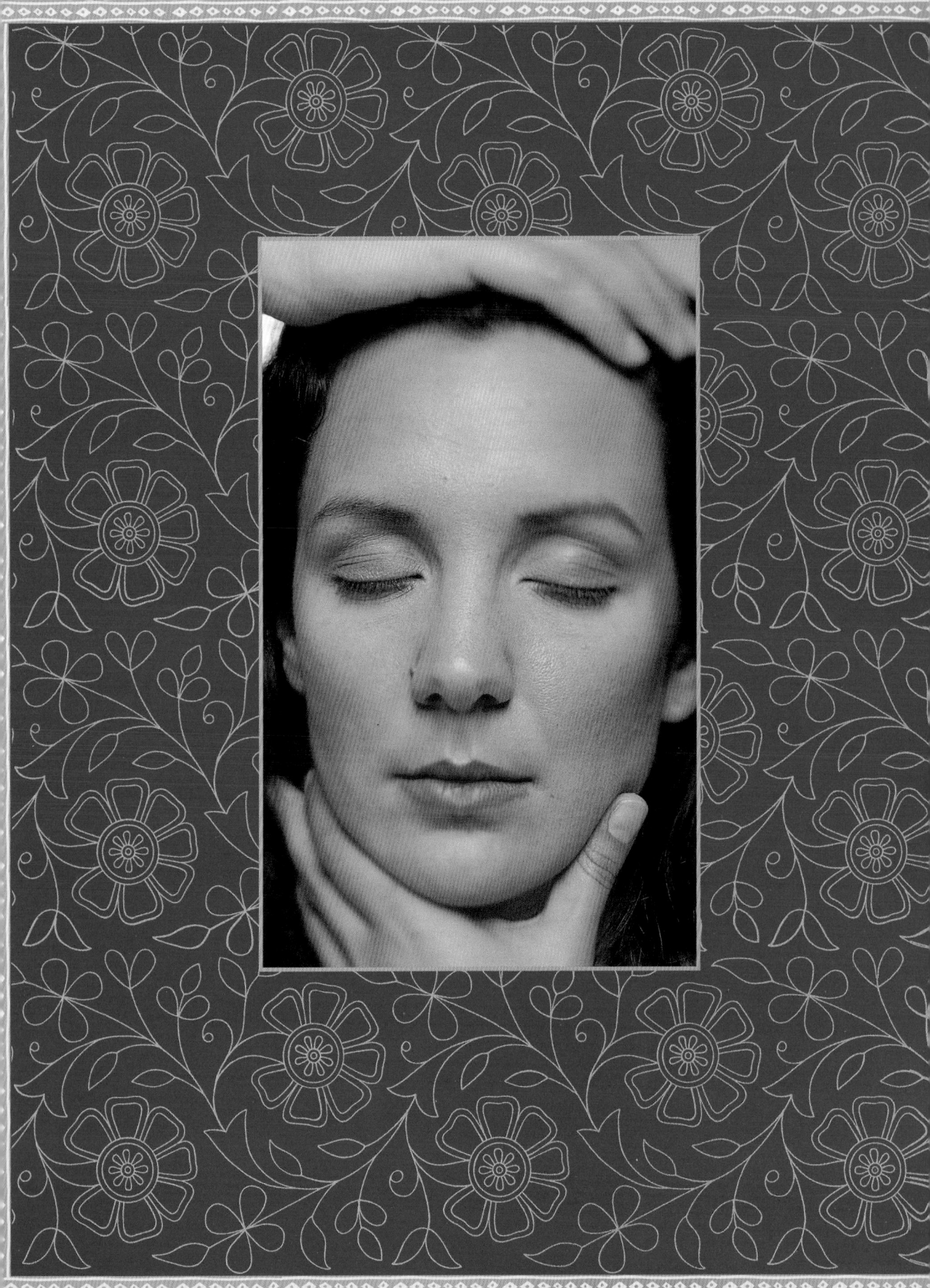

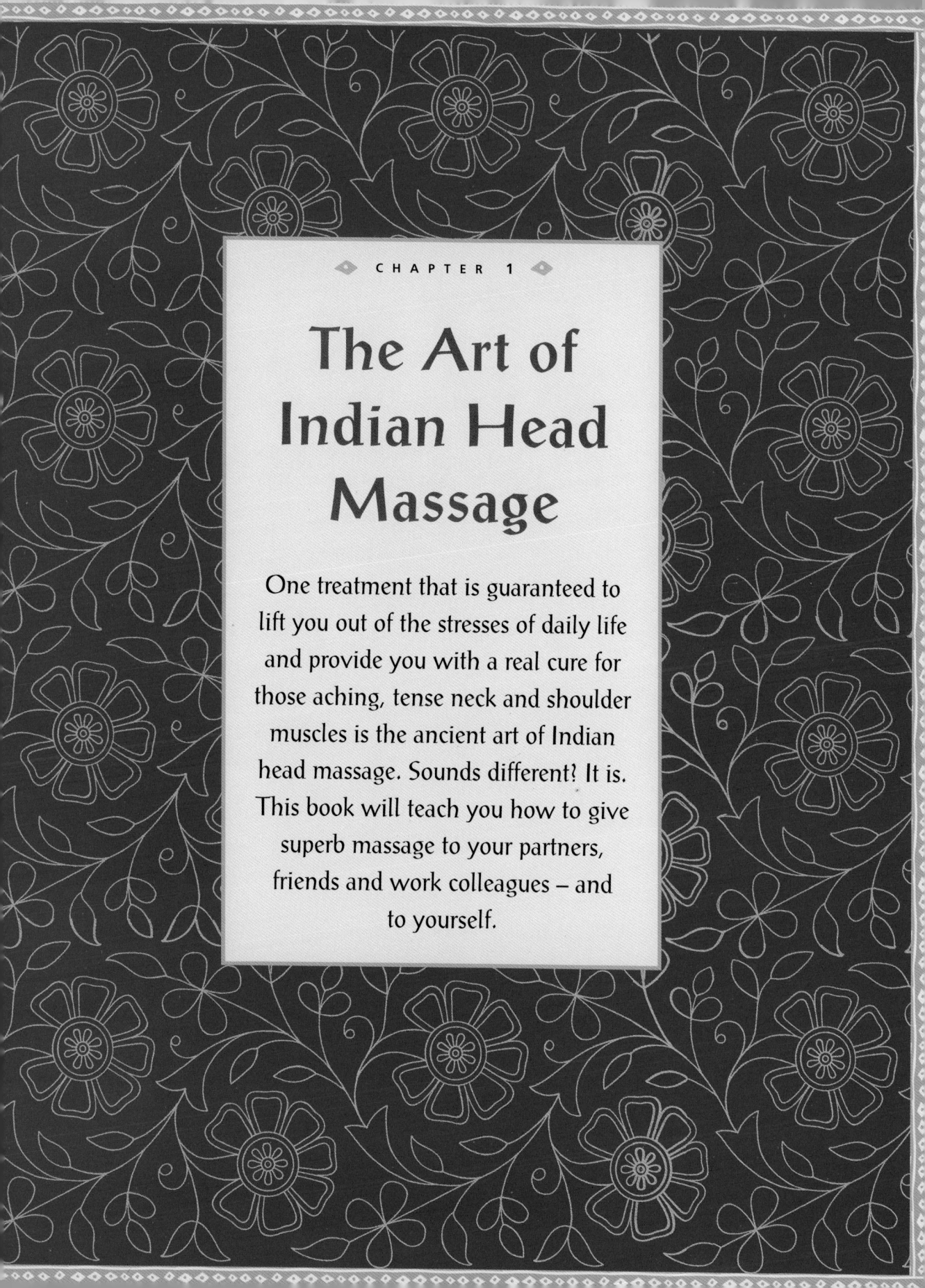

# CHAPTER 1

# The Art of Indian Head Massage

One treatment that is guaranteed to lift you out of the stresses of daily life and provide you with a real cure for those aching, tense neck and shoulder muscles is the ancient art of Indian head massage. Sounds different? It is. This book will teach you how to give superb massage to your partners, friends and work colleagues – and to yourself.

# INTRODUCTION

You are a very special person if you can boast immunity to the pressures of modern-day living. Those who fall prey to stress often complain that tension is stored in the shoulder, neck and head areas. Indian head massage is guaranteed to relieve these feelings. The technique has been practised in India for over a thousand years, originally by women who believed that massaging their heads with natural vegetable oils kept their long hair healthy and strong. They were right. Massaging the scalp stimulates the flow of blood to the follicles, improving the supply of nutrients needed for healthy hair growth. Nowadays the most common cause of poor blood flow is stress-generated muscle tension. By helping to dispel such tension, head massage not only improves the condition of your hair, but also provides an invaluable treatment for stress-linked problems like headaches and eyestrain.

# WHAT IS INDIAN HEAD MASSAGE?

The traditional Indian head massage practised by women in India was restricted to the head and hair. However, I have extended the techniques to include the neck, shoulders and upper arms. Indian head massage is a safe, simple, yet effective therapy that not only promotes hair growth, but also provides relief from aches and pains. It is renowned for relieving symptoms of stress. Now you can learn these new techniques, which combine an ancient cultural tradition with the demands of modern living, to use at home.

# How Does it Work?

The head, neck and shoulders are important energy centres within your body. If you are feeling stressed or angry, tension tends to accumulate. This tension can later show up as a stiff neck and shoulders, eye strain and sometimes even hair loss. Indian head massage involves working with a firm and gentle rhythm to help unknot blockages and relieve this uncomfortable build-up of tension. However, its effect is not just physical: it works on an emotional level too, calming the spirit, promoting relaxation and relieving stress.

An ancient proverb states: 'A happy mind is medicine; no better prescription exists.' I have found results bear this out. People who come to my clinic feeling despondent, depressed, worried, tense, stressed and distressed leave in a happier and more relaxed frame of mind after just one soothing Indian head massage.

'Regular head massage is wonderfully relaxing, enhances the health of the scalp and promotes the growth of lustrous hair.' The Observer

Indian head massage offers the means by which the individual can begin to get in touch with the healing potential within the hitherto unexplored regions of their inner being and thus become empowered to ensure their own well-being.

# THE HISTORY OF INDIAN HEAD MASSAGE

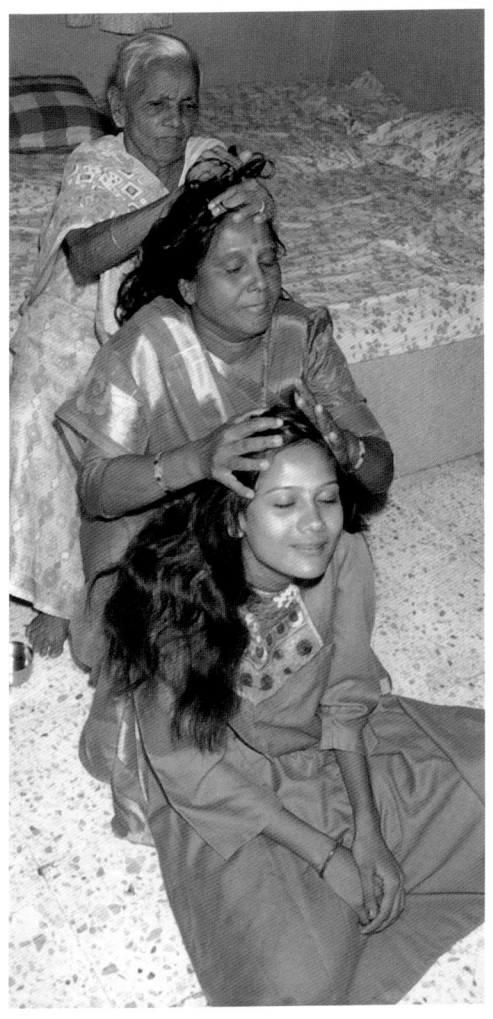

Massage has always played an important part in Indian life, featuring in the earliest Ayurvedic texts that date back nearly 4,000 years. When used in conjunction with herbs, spices and aromatic oils, massage had an important medical function and could not only 'strengthen muscles and firm the skin', but also encourage the body's natural healing abilities. Today, Indian infants still often receive a daily massage from birth to keep them in good health. From three to six years old, they are massaged once or twice a week, and after the age of six, they are taught to share a massage with family members on a regular basis. Massage then occurs across the generations as an integral part of family life. My own family is typical of many others in this respect.

Indian head massage springs from this rich tradition of intergenerational family massage, and has been practised for over a thousand years. It was originally developed by women as a part of their grooming routine. They used different oils according to the season (coconut, sesame, almond, olive oil, herbal oils, buttermilk, mustard oil and henna) to keep their hair strong, lustrous and in beautiful condition.

The benefits of head massage were not confined exclusively to women: barbers practised many of these same skills. They used to ply their trade by going to individuals' houses, cutting men's hair and offering 'champi' (head massage) as part of the treatment. In time, this became quite a custom: everyone, including royalty, would receive regular head massage from their own barber. Treatments differed from the massages performed by women in that the barbers were mainly giving invigorating scalp massages designed primarily to stimulate and refresh the individual, rather than to care for the hair. Echoes of this Indian tradition reached the West long before the practice itself in the form of the word 'shampoo', which comes from the Hindi word 'champi'. Being 'champi-ed' meant having your head massaged.

Massage skills have evolved through the ages and have been handed down from barber father to barber son in much the same way that the women in the family have kept the tradition of hair massage and grooming by passing it down from mother to daughter right up to the present day. In India nowadays, it is very common to go to

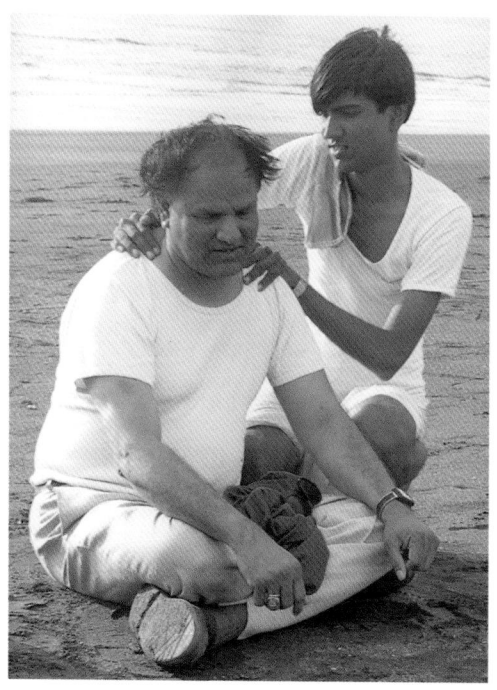

a barber's shop, receive a wet shave or haircut and have a head massage thrown in as part of the treatment. A word of warning: should you experience one of these massages in India, do ask your barber not to click your neck, which is a normal part of their head massage. Head massage can now also be seen in many other locations in India: on street corners, at markets and on the beach ... so you can even experience a wonderfully relaxing Indian head massage with the rising or setting sun for company!

# The Development of Indian Head Massage

Like most of my compatriots, I grew up with head massage as an integral part of my daily life. As a child, my mother would give me a head massage with coconut oil and, as I grew older, it was something to be automatically experienced every time I visited a barber. I came to England to train as a physiotherapist in the 70s but was disappointed to find that the massage element of this discipline was being neglected. I then took a course in full-body massage and, not surprisingly, was still not taught any techniques involving the head. I was dismayed to discover that massage always stopped at the neck and nobody practised head massage – not even full-body massage therapists. No one had shown them how!

I began to miss the therapeutic value of regular head massage and decided that I wanted to bring this therapy to the West. Experience had taught me that head massage could bring tremendous relief from aches and pains, not only in the head, but also in other parts of the body. Knowing this, I decided to introduce a system of massage to this country that would encompass the head and upper neck and bring relief to the many who suffer from aches and pains in those previously neglected areas.

In 1978, I decided to return to India and research head massage wherever it was practised. In centres as far apart as Calcutta and Bombay, in the cities and in the countryside, simple head massage is widespread. Barbers in barber shops perform this service for their clients, you can find it on street corners, beaches and in family homes. However, although I enjoyed being worked on, I couldn't help feeling that there was something missing in the massage. This type of simple massage does not get to the deep-rooted source of stress. So, although there was some improvement in my well-being following these head massages, the effects were too short-lived.

During my experiments with head massage in India, I found that the methods used varied from person to person. The barbers would concentrate on my scalp, while my mother and her women friends focused on treating the hair. In addition, everyone who worked with me had his or her own individual technique, which had been handed down and developed through the generations. I decided that I would begin to formalize what I was experiencing and use the knowledge of my massage training to discover which part of my body reacted most positively to various moves. Because of my blindness, my other senses have become very finely tuned and I was able to concentrate with complete absorption on the effect the massage was having. By this means, I was able to devise a therapy that would bring the greatest relief to the multitude of problems concentrated in the head. I soon concluded that the therapy would benefit by being extended to include not only the head, but also the neck, shoulders and upper arms.

Having formalized the techniques of Indian head massage, I wanted to pass the knowledge on to others. In 1981, while I was thinking about how to introduce this idea to the public, a friend suggested that I take a stand at the Mind, Body, Spirit exhibition at Olympia in London. By the end of the exhibition, over 170 people suffering from exhibition exhaustion, headaches and work-related stress had tried it out. They felt relaxed and recharged. Some people even attended more than once.

My experience at the exhibition built up my confidence. I gained a great deal of experience in different types of hair and hair styles and I explored ways of revising my techniques to include massage that was suitable for every type of hair.

The exhibition led to a wave of publicity and numerous magazine articles. As a result, many more people became interested in learning and practising Indian head massage. This gave me the idea of arranging courses, and the more successful of these were the weekend courses. These enabled me to teach my pupils slowly and allowed time for revision. These weekend courses continued with great success up until 1995. From 1995 I introduced a course which led to a qualification to practise head massage. This included weekend instruction plus home study, case studies and an exam so that I could recommend the qualified therapists to anyone with confidence. These courses are still continuing and remain extremely popular.

Over the years at my clinic and at various exhibitions countless clients have allowed me to study the effect of my techniques in depth and to develop and expand them. One of the most important developments in my techniques was the introduction of an Ayurvedic element of chakra energy balancing and the extension of the massage element to include massage of the face and ears to enhance the overall effect.

Ayurveda is an ancient Indian medical system, which some believe to be the oldest medical system in the world. It goes beyond the limits of 'healing', placing an emphasis on balance and the uniqueness of each individual. Within Ayurveda, as in other belief systems from around the world, the body is said to contain seven energy centres. The energy points are known by different names in different parts of the world: I shall call them chakras. The flow of energy around the body and through these centres is believed to have a great effect on a person's well-being.

Once I had incorporated an Ayurvedic element, I found I had a powerful therapy to increase the physical, mental and subtle energy benefits of Indian head massage. I call this therapy Indian Champissage. Champissage goes beyond simple Indian head massage. It combines physical massage with a more subtle form of massage which affects a person's energy centres. The chakras I concentrate on in my work are the three higher chakras: Sahasrara located on the crown of the head, Ajna – vision (the third eye) – located in the middle of the forehead and Vishuddha, located in the throat. In total there are seven chakras, but they do not work independently of each other. A dysfunction in any one of them will result in a knock-on effect, which will ultimately build up and spiral to the head, culminating in a feeling of stress and tension. Working on the higher chakras has a powerful effect, and can bring the energy of the whole body back into balance. This cannot be realized through simple massage and is unique to Champissage.

# The Seven Chakras

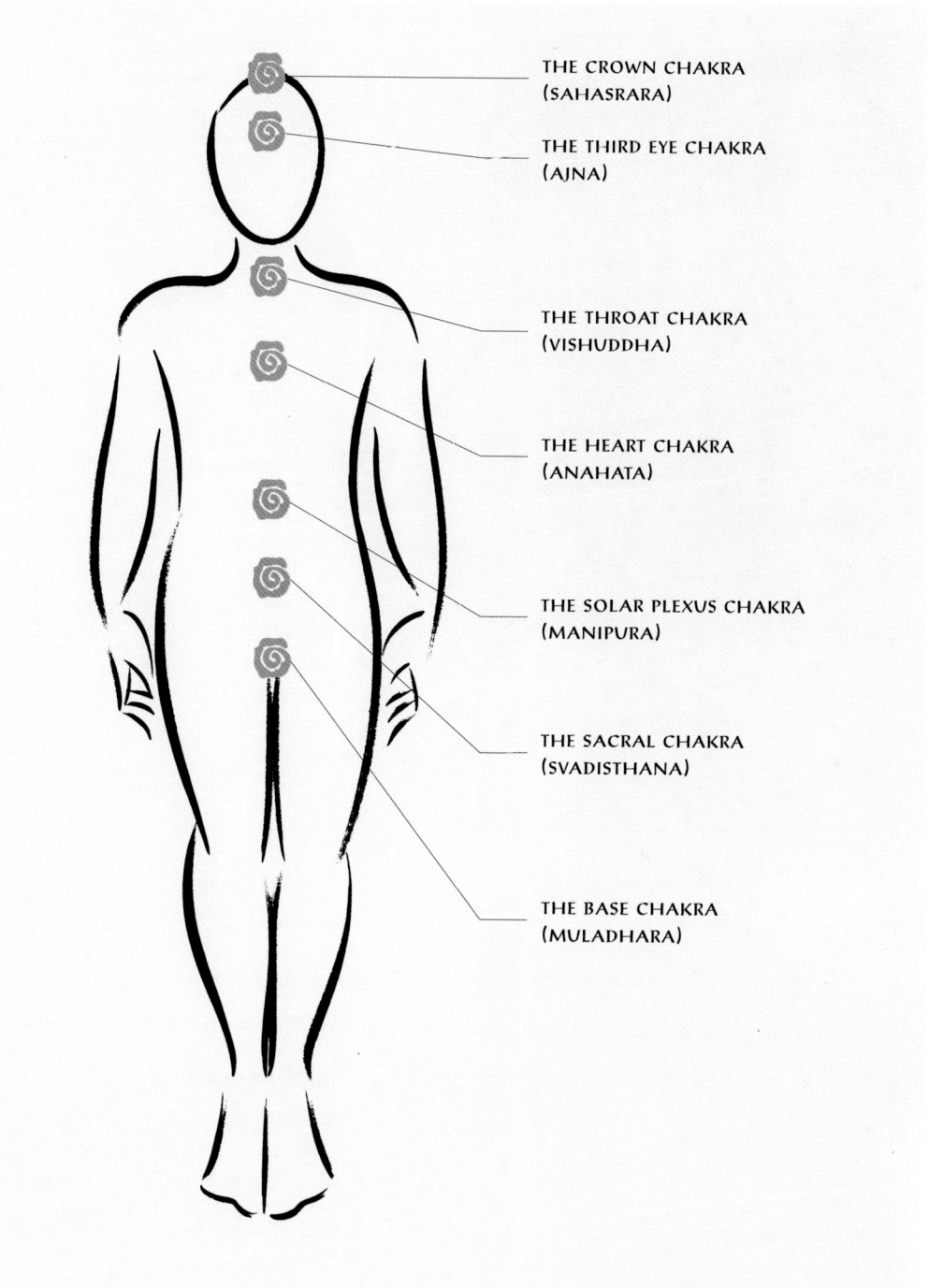

THE CROWN CHAKRA
(SAHASRARA)

THE THIRD EYE CHAKRA
(AJNA)

THE THROAT CHAKRA
(VISHUDDHA)

THE HEART CHAKRA
(ANAHATA)

THE SOLAR PLEXUS CHAKRA
(MANIPURA)

THE SACRAL CHAKRA
(SVADISTHANA)

THE BASE CHAKRA
(MULADHARA)

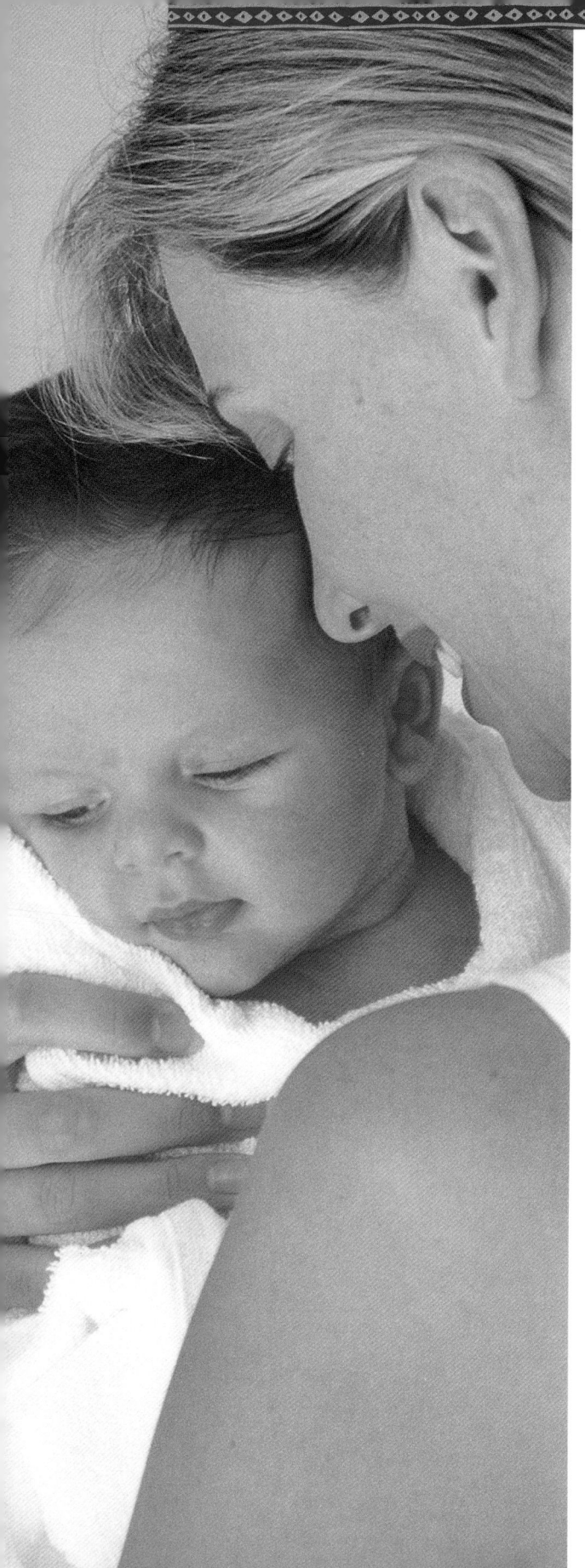

# THE POWER OF TOUCH

Amongst higher animals, touch and grooming form an important part of daily life. Many hours are spent in these activities, which provide comfort and create close social bonds. As highly evolved primates, touch remains a fundamental part of our biological heritage and plays a vital role in our development from infants to adults.

As babies, our most powerful experiences come through the medium of touch. We reach out to touch and explore the world around us, and we are also held and cradled by our parents. Many studies have shown that the quality and amount of handling that a young baby receives is crucial for healthy physical, emotional and mental development. For example, groups of baby rats that were handled and stroked with gentleness and care grew up to have greater body weight and brain size, less fear of the external world, and an increased resistance to stress and disease compared to groups of rats that were infrequently and roughly handled.

A famous study conducted by Harlow on Rhesus monkeys in America goes even further in demonstrating the primary importance of touch. In the experiment, infant monkeys raised in the laboratory were given a choice of two surrogate mothers. One was made of soft terry cloth and lit from behind with a light bulb for warmth. The other mother was made of wire mesh, but possessed an artificial nipple which supplied milk. Time and again the monkeys clung to the terry-cloth 'mother' for comfort rather than the milk-providing 'mother'. Only when the infants were extremely hungry would they be forced to make a brief dash for milk, scampering back to the comfort mother afterwards.

This experiment also demonstrated how important touch is to healthy personality development and social skills. These laboratory-raised monkeys were introduced to other monkeys of similar age but were totally unable to co-exist peacefully with them. Furthermore, when it came to raising baby monkeys themselves, the laboratory monkeys demonstrated no maternal attachment.

Touch is essential for stimulating our nervous system and promoting healthy physical development. However, it is also critical for our mental and social development. A large part of our self-definition and the way we feel about ourselves comes from the way we are held and touched by our parents. Through it we develop a sense of being valued and of being valuable which is the cornerstone of our self-esteem. We learn about pleasure, warmth and comfort from touch. We learn about expressing our feelings, we learn about reassurance and security, and we learn about connectedness and social bonding.

Children who come from families where there is insufficient physical contact and tenderness may find it difficult to accept and value themselves. They may have difficulty expressing themselves emotionally, and find it hard to form long-term, intimate relationships as adults.

## Touch connects us to the outside world, brings people closer and weaves intimacy

## INTERNATIONAL TOUCH

In the same way that some families are more touch-friendly than others, some national cultures are more touch or physically orientated than others. In one study of the number of physical interactions that occurred during one hour in cafes, the highest number of recorded incidents occurred in Puerto Rico with a staggering 180 in one hour. This contrasted with a despondent zero in London! It is difficult to isolate the separate influence of family and cultural background, but they must combine to have an impact on how we relate physically to other people.

Touch is an instinctive, natural language that we all speak and understand. It is from this instinctive language of rubbing, holding and comforting that more structured forms of touch have evolved to eventually develop into the different forms of massage that exist in every culture throughout the world. English people are traditionally very reserved and puritanical when it comes to being touched. One of the wonderful things about massage is that it is a formalized touch; it gives you license to touch someone within established and defined boundaries.

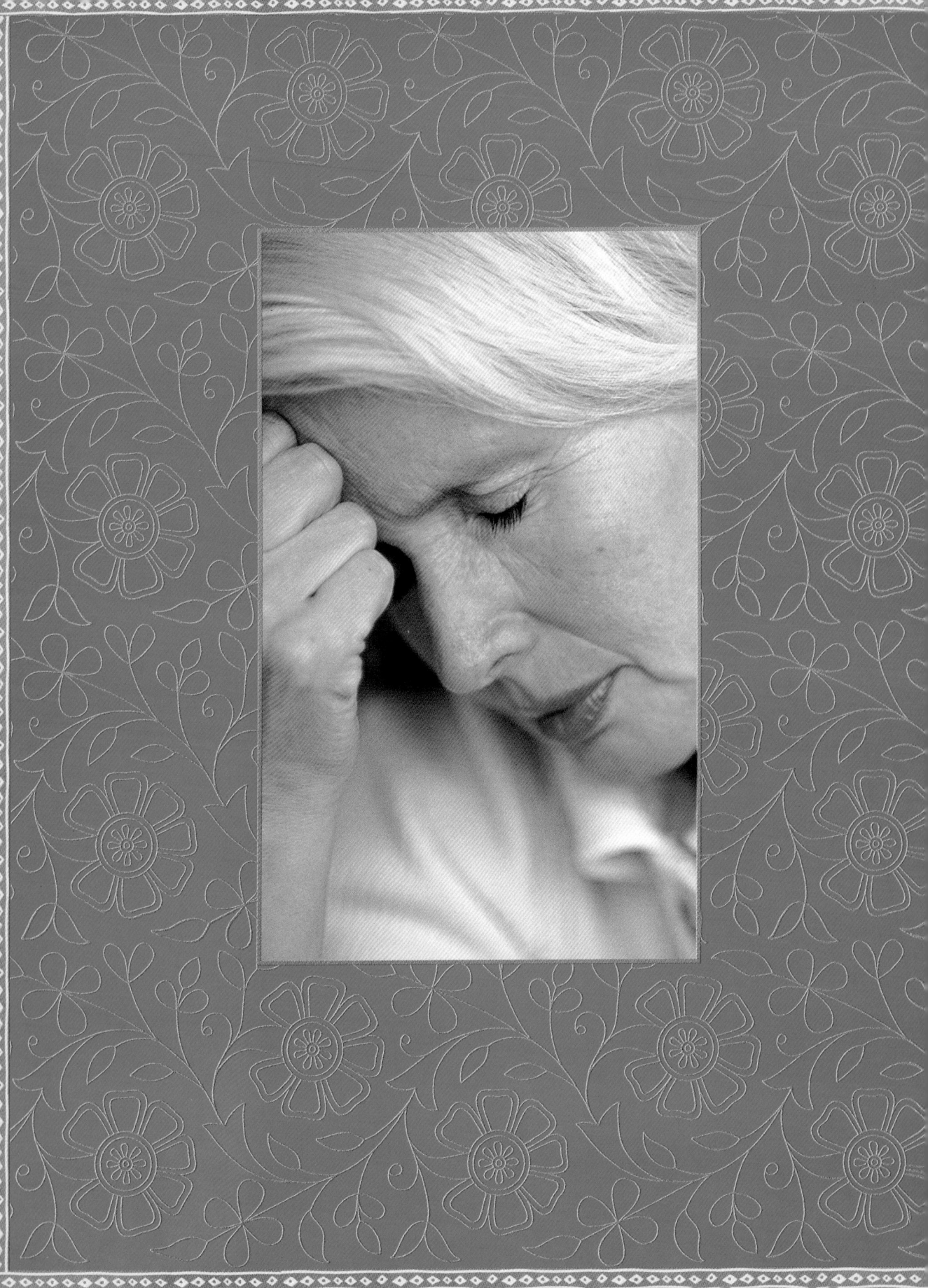

# CHAPTER 2

# Managing Stress

What is stress? Does just getting
up in the morning make you feel
stressed? How do you feel right now?
If I were to mention the word exam,
or traffic jam, redundancy, deadline
or tax demand, how would you feel
then? Beginning to feel just a little
stressed out? Then read on.

# INTRODUCTION

The dictionary defines stress as a constraining or impelling force, effort or demand upon physical or mental energy. A stressor is a person or situation that makes you become stressed.

We in the modern world are far more likely to suffer from the effects of stress than our ancestors were. Seventy percent of all illness is now directly attributed to stress. Modern society with its pressures, overcrowding, traffic congestion, noise, fears and general uncertainties regarding work, home and family life, tends to present situation upon situation in which the possibility of becoming stressed is ever present. Stress is an unavoidable part of modern life: everyone experiences stress and everyday stresses are not

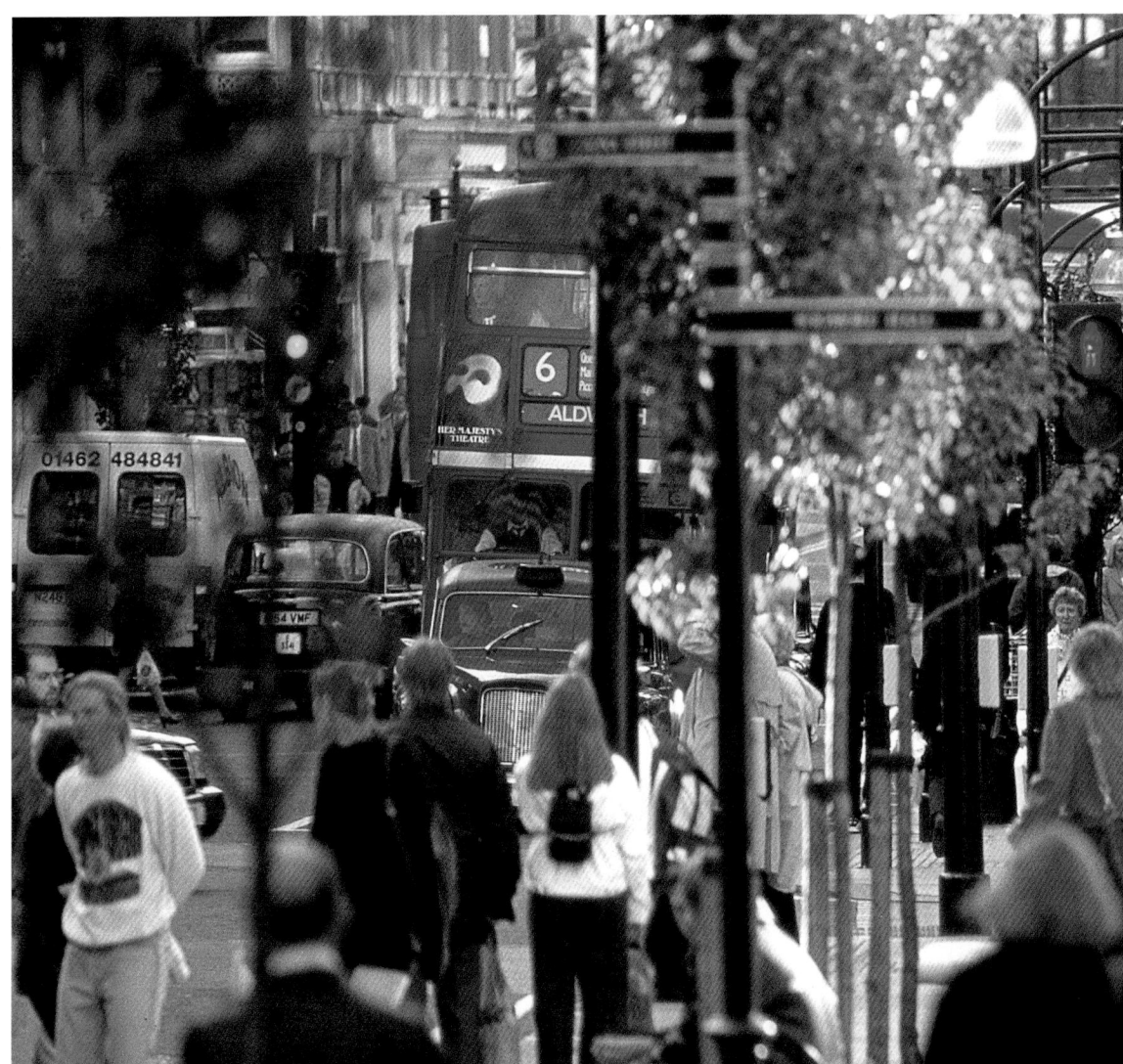

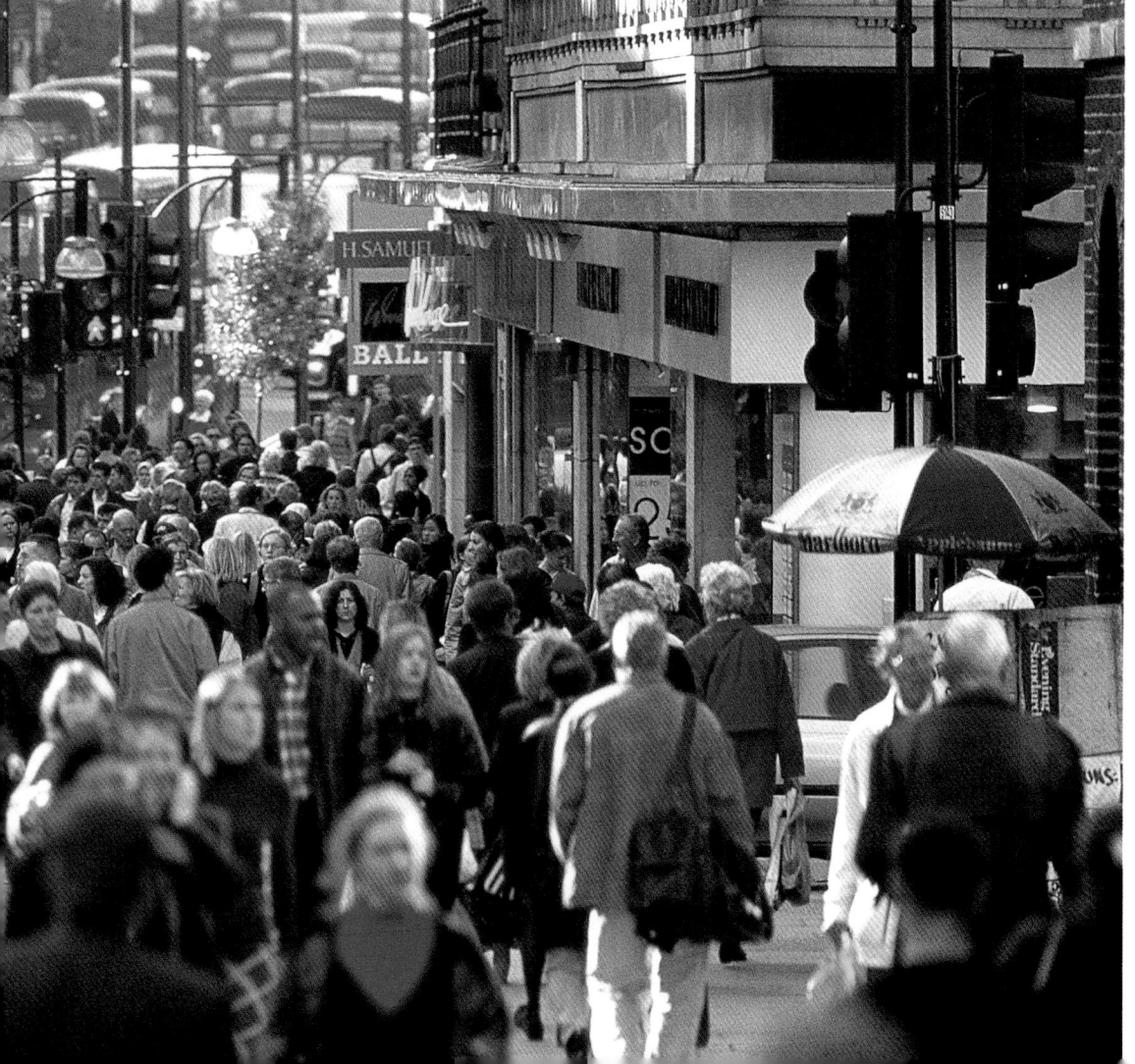

necessarily harmful. In fact, stress is not always negative but can often be just stimulating enough to make life enjoyable, or at least interesting. If you want to compete and excel in sports, for example, you need stress to bring about the motivation to perform. Some people handle stress very well while others are more negatively influenced by it. It is the effect of long-term stress that can be positively harmful to our bodies.

It may seem strange that your body is capable of damaging itself at all, but this chapter will show you how the body responds to perceived threat, and how those responses can become harmful when they are not dealt with appropriately.

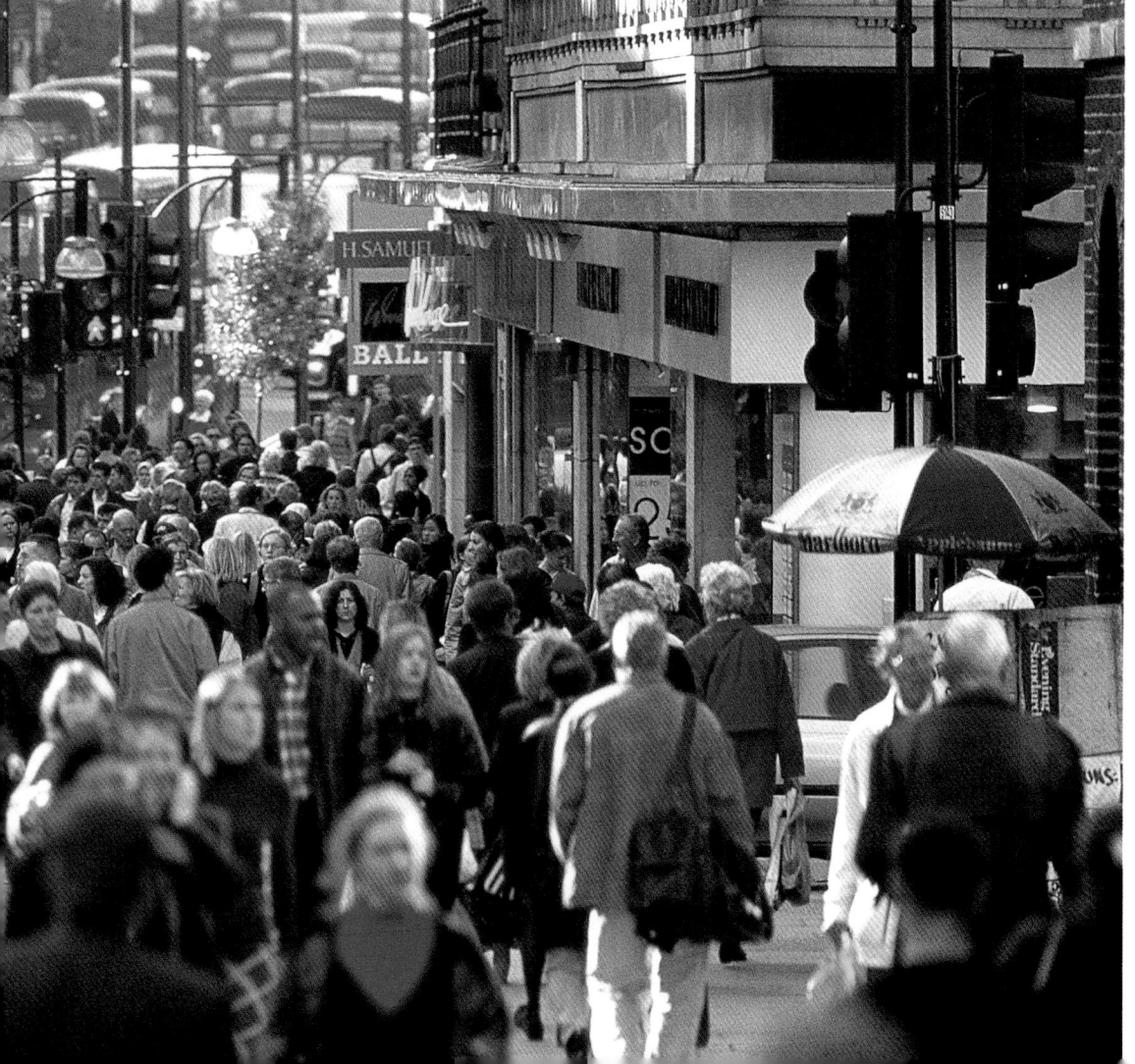

# WHAT CAUSES STRESS?

So, if stress can be good for us, when do stress levels become harmful? The factors that seem to make any situation dangerously stressful are:

- Lack of predictability
- Lack of control
- Lack of outlets for frustration

When these elements are present, even innocuous situations can become stressful and produce a reaction that is completely out of proportion to the cause. It comes down to the fact that it's not the situation but our reaction to it that creates the stress in our lives. Our fears and anxieties about past events repeating themselves add to the vicious circle, and the uncertainties of life crowd our mind with frightening possibilities.

## CASE HISTORY

Age: 37
Sex: Male
Profession: Small business owner

- Symptoms: Carlos came to my clinic suffering from upper back pain. He was anxious and depressed – chiefly because of the constant pain. When Carlos was thirteen, he had had a bad riding accident. Stress and the pressure of running a small business had exacerbated his back problem.
- After the first treatment: He felt a little dizzy (this is normal) but very mellow. His upper back was still aching. I advised him that, for something to get better, there often has to be a period of transition when the pain almost seems worse. However, the following day Carlos noticed a considerable decrease in the pain.
- After subsequent treatments: He felt spaced out, but in a nice way. His back problem was no longer a cause for concern because he no longer suffered from pain.
- Further recommendations: To attend my clinic once a fortnight for a month, then once a month for a further three months.

As human beings we have a tendency to focus on the past and the future and withdraw our attention from the present moment. Yet it is in the present moment that we have the greatest clarity to deal with any situation. Life is a journey and enjoying it can replace the holding back and the holding on which in turn create fear and ultimately stress. Struggle begins almost at birth and we must not forget that positive lessons can be learned through adversity. If you or I truly knew what stretched out before us there would be no growth.

Growth is usually preceded by change. However, handling change can be difficult in the short term and the following life-changing events have been identified as the most likely to cause negative or harmful stress:

- Bereavement
- Moving house
- Debt
- Ill health
- Difficult relationships
- Stressful work
- Family problems

Even positive events, such as a marriage, pregnancy or a child starting school or university may cause you stress, and may ultimately lead to illness. In war, which is a state of extremely heightened and continual stress, front-line soldiers will eventually go into shell shock or battle fatigue if kept under fire for too long, and the same is true of our daily struggles. But remember that your personality and coping-mechanisms will largely determine how you deal with these daily stresses and strains. Now you have a very important ally in the battle against stress: Indian head massage!

# How Your Body Reacts to Stress

When someone is subjected to stress, input from the five senses travels through the nervous system and triggers the hypothalamus in the brain to send out signals. These signals reach the pituitary gland, which is the master gland of the endocrine system. A hormonal response sent from the pituitary gland triggers the adrenal glands to release adrenaline into the bloodstream to prepare the body for 'fight or flight'.

The normal functioning of the body is disrupted, as a body in a state of stress needs to conserve its energy to propel muscles. The adrenaline coursing through the bloodstream causes blood pressure to rise and muscles to tense. Breathing becomes shallow and rapid, sexual desire and hunger are suppressed and digestion stops. The brain becomes hyper-alert.

As a temporary expedient, the stress response is vital, but if the situation is prolonged, with no release of tension, the result can be disastrous. As well as increasing the heart rate and the blood pressure, the body also diverts vital resources from the immune system and cholesterol levels rise. Common symptoms of prolonged stress include fatigue, headache, heartburn, indigestion, hair loss, insomnia and depression.

Some more serious conditions and diseases associated with prolonged stress are acidosis, backache, Irritable Bowel Syndrome, Crohn's disease, diverticulosis, pancreatic and kidney disease and even heart attacks.

'Regular [head] massage helps people work better. Absenteeism through stress would drop immediately if everyone had a massage at least once a week.' Daily Mail

## Do You Recognize this Person?

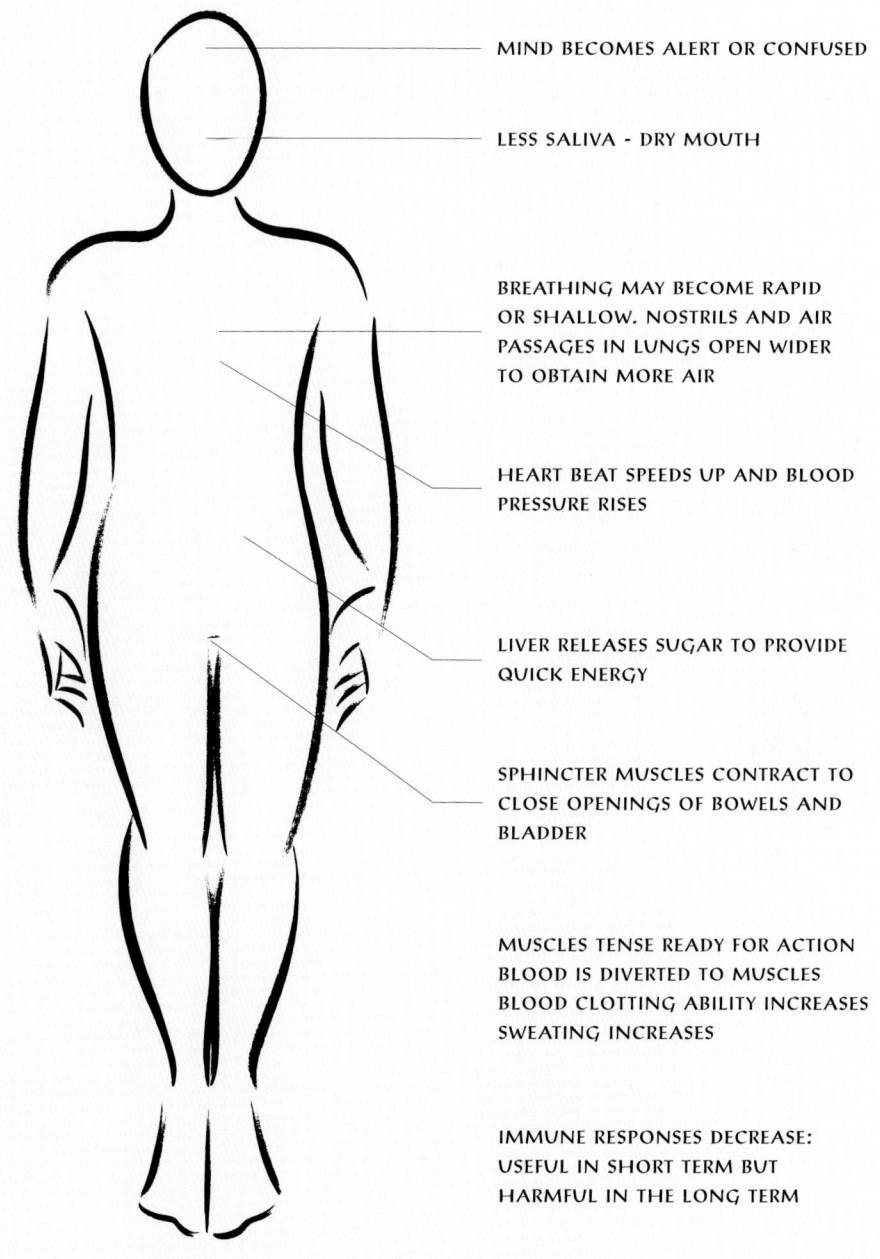

MIND BECOMES ALERT OR CONFUSED

LESS SALIVA - DRY MOUTH

BREATHING MAY BECOME RAPID
OR SHALLOW. NOSTRILS AND AIR
PASSAGES IN LUNGS OPEN WIDER
TO OBTAIN MORE AIR

HEART BEAT SPEEDS UP AND BLOOD
PRESSURE RISES

LIVER RELEASES SUGAR TO PROVIDE
QUICK ENERGY

SPHINCTER MUSCLES CONTRACT TO
CLOSE OPENINGS OF BOWELS AND
BLADDER

MUSCLES TENSE READY FOR ACTION
BLOOD IS DIVERTED TO MUSCLES
BLOOD CLOTTING ABILITY INCREASES
SWEATING INCREASES

IMMUNE RESPONSES DECREASE:
USEFUL IN SHORT TERM BUT
HARMFUL IN THE LONG TERM

# RECOGNIZING THE SIGNS

Although your body's reaction to stress, described on the previous page, may sound drastic, we don't always realize immediately when we are suffering from stress. There are several physical symptoms that can act as warning signals: advance notice from our body telling us to take preemptive action. Check the following list. The more symptoms you have, the more pressure your body is under.

◆ Shallow and/or faster breathing

◆ High blood pressure/palpitations

◆ Excess sweating

◆ Muscular tension

◆ Dilated pupils

◆ Loss of appetite

◆ Irregular menstruation

◆ Impotence

◆ Low sex drive

◆ Ulcers

◆ Constipation

◆ Diarrhoea

◆ Hair loss

◆ Constant tiredness

◆ PMT

◆ Disturbed sleeping pattern

◆ Poor skin

◆ Poor hair condition

As well as experiencing one or more of the physical symptoms listed above, the emotions can also be thrown into turmoil. Anyone under a lot of stress will feel uneasy and vulnerable and may feel like crying continually. It is common to feel overwhelmed by negative emotions and to simply feel unable to cope with life. Different people react to these feelings in different ways but they can sometimes lead to violent behaviour or reliance on alcohol or drugs. The important thing is to recognize that these symptoms are the result of stress and to tackle the underlying cause.

Emotional disturbance can surface in many ways. The following is a checklist of feelings commonly experienced when under a lot of stress.

- Feelings of helplessness
- Loneliness
- Panic attacks
- Irritability
- Desire to escape
- Frustration
- Mood swings
- Insecurity
- Anxiety
- Over-stimulation
- Loss of sense of humour
- Low self-esteem
- Nightmares
- Lack of concentration
- Confusion
- Loss of sense of proportion
- Forgetfulness
- Hypochondria
- Phobias

When the physical, mental and emotional bodies are out of balance we need assistance to restore comfort and harmony. A sense of peace, tranquillity and wholeness can then ensue.

Indian head massage is an ideal way to restore homeostasis. Whilst giving Indian head massage, I can truly say that every person gives me positive feedback. So much peace is restored within each person that I am supremely confident that Indian head massage is a perfect tool to deal with the results of stress. The massage tackles the physical, mental and emotional effects of stress in a unique and particularly effective way.

'If you are distressed by anything external, the pain is not due to the thing itself but to your estimate of it.' Marcus Aurelius

# STRESS IN THE WORKPLACE

Tackling stress effectively is especially important in the workplace. Each year several million working days are lost as a result of stress. Two out of three medical consultations concern stress-related conditions.

Stress is not only caused by a high-pressure job; anyone can succumb: from the managing director to the office cleaner. We spend a major part of our lives at work, or looking for it. Thus, what happens at work is vitally important to our health and well-being. Stress can occur if you are working in an environment or a job that is not really right for you, or if you feel that your abilities are being over or under stretched. Your section leader or your boss may not appreciate your personal attributes, or strained personal relationships may begin to have an extremely negative effect on you.

## CASE HISTORY

Age: 20
Sex: Female
Profession: Student

◆ Symptoms: Although Lillian complained of acne and dark circles under her eyes, the real problem was that she had lost the ability to concentrate. She was very worried about the approaching exams but her lethargic state prevented her from doing anything about it. She decided to try Indian head massage as a last resort.
◆ After the first treatment: Her neck and shoulders, which had been as stiff as boards, opened up. She felt like a new person and because the stored-up, tense energy had been shifted she felt able to return to her flat and get down to some real study.
◆ After subsequent treatments: Lillian found she couldn't keep her eyes open during the sessions! She became much less stressed, her skin tone improved, the dark circles under her eyes disappeared and her smile returned. She was able to tackle her exams with confidence and she decided to tell her all her friends about Indian head massage.
◆ Further recommendations: I suggested that Lillian should drink plenty of water, exercise daily and eat good, wholesome food, if possible avoiding the standard student fare of junk food.

Your physical working conditions can also cause stress: a noisy office, working in a factory all day, sitting at a VDU screen, bad lighting and insufficient working space can all take their toll on your health and well-being.

Check out the following situations. Have any of them affected your performance at work?

- Trapped in an unsatisfying job
- Lack of feedback
- Inadequate rewards – low salary
- Poor prospects
- Threat of redundancy
- Deadlines
- Changes in working practice requiring new skills
- Responsibility without adequate authority
- Geographic relocation
- Lack of stimulation at work
- Unsympathetic boss
- Hostile clients, customers and work colleagues
- Frequent night shifts

You're not alone! According to the Confederation of British Industry (CBI), illness caused by stress in the workplace has increased by 500% since the mid 1950s. Fortunately, there is something you can do about it whenever you feel one or more of the symptoms of stress creeping up on you.

If stress in the workplace is properly managed it can be re-experienced as a motivator. Indian head massage is well suited to the corporate environment because of its flexible and portable nature and the fact that the treatment is quick and the recipient does not need to undress. No creams, oils or special equipment are used. It is a time-saving therapy when time is of the essence because the therapist can come to you. When I see clients in the workplace, the treatment is quick (just 15 to 20 minutes) and easy to perform. It is therefore perfect for the office where time is precious.

## Office Exercises

If you are one of the growing army of office workers in the West, then this exercise workout is especially designed for you. These de-stressing exercises are simple to perform and you don't have to leave your office or even your desk to try them.

This unique workout will take no more than 8 to 10 minutes. It can be fitted in at any time during your working day, no matter how busy you think you may be. Although being outside in the fresh air or regular visits to the gym are the best ways to exercise, these options are not always available in the high-powered office culture of the 90s. With long working hours, tight deadlines and job insecurity, it is difficult to make exercise a priority. But it is certain that without exercise you will start to feel the effects of stress and you will find that you are less able to cope with everyday pressure. Your mental and physical health will start to suffer.

Fitting this workout into your office routine is the next best thing to visiting a gym for relieving tension, helping you to relax and correcting your posture. It will also help your concentration, enabling you to perform your work more efficiently throughout the day. Try doing this workout during your coffee or lunch break, or whenever you feel tired or that you just can't cope. These exercises will give your mind a workout, as well as your body, making you feel more alert. In addition to this workout, try to start cutting down on tea and coffee, replacing them with mineral water. It is a good idea to have a large bottle of water on your desk to sip from whenever you feel like it and to try to finish the bottle by the end of the day. The combination of these exercises and the effects of less caffeine will mean you will notice a real difference in your body and mood within two to three weeks.

## BEFORE YOU START

◆ Sit straight on a chair with your shoulders held back, hands on your lap, both feet on the ground.

◆ Repeat all the exercises three times. Do not strain. Breathe in when carrying out each exercise and breathe out when releasing it.

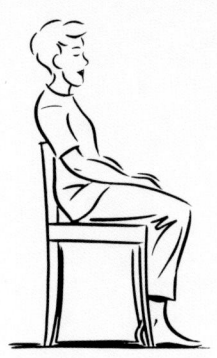

## NECK STRETCH (SEE ILLUSTRATIONS)

This will relieve tension from the neck and improve mobility.

1   Sit looking straight ahead and then gently bring your head towards your chest as far as it will go. Hold for three seconds and return to the starting position. Repeat.
2   Gently bring your head back as far as you can and hold for three seconds then release. Repeat.
3   Bring your head towards the left shoulder, keeping your right shoulder down, hold for five seconds then release. Repeat.
4   Repeat on the right side.
5   Look towards your left shoulder as far as possible without moving your body. Hold for three seconds then release.
6   Repeat on the right side.

NECK STRETCH 1

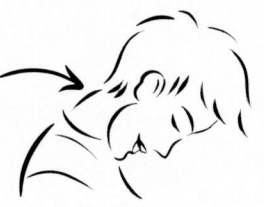

NECK STRETCH 2

## SHOULDER LIFT

This shoulder exercise releases muscular tension and increases the mobility of the shoulders while improving posture.

1   Take a deep breath and at the same time lift both shoulders as high as possible.
2   Hold for three seconds then breathe out and release.
3   Repeat.

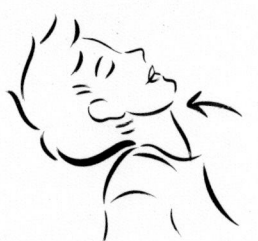

NECK STRETCH 3

## ARM STRETCH

1   Breathe in, stretch your arms out to the sides and shake your wrists and fingers.
2   Breathe out and let your arms fall by your sides.
3   Repeat.
4   Now breathe in and raise your arms to the ceiling.
5   Breathe out and release.

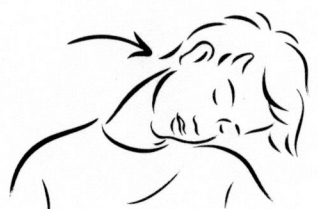

NECK STRETCH 5

## EYE REST

This is an excellent exercise for relieving eye strain and tension headaches.

1   Resting your elbows on the desk, cover your face and eyes with your hands.
2   Make sure you don't hunch your shoulders up: try to keep them down and relaxed.
3   Keeping your eyes and mouth closed, take three slow, deep breaths, breathing in and out only through your nose.

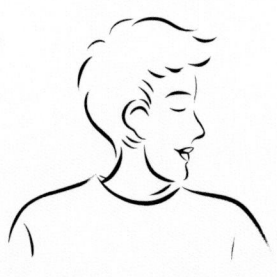

## Mental Relaxation Exercise

The following exercise relaxes you mentally and will be of great help as an addition to the physical exercises above. You will find that it helps to calm down your busy mind, improving your concentration and making you more focused.

This short meditation exercise will clear your mind of all stress and tension. Sit comfortably with your head level, eyes to the front. Close your eyes and focus on your breathing. Breathe slowly and rhythmically. Always try to breathe in and out through your nose. Breathe deeply, using the diaphragm and allowing your ribcage to expand and relax. Sit straight with your shoulders back and down and both feet on the ground.

Now imagine that you are in one of your favourite places. Savour the colours, sounds and aromas around you. Relax and enjoy the soothing environment. Your body and mind will begin feel calm and refreshed. Stay in this position for five to ten minutes.

Only when you are ready, slowly open your eyes. Stretch your arms, first at shoulder level, then above your head. You should be able to return to this meditation at will.

CASE HISTORY

Age: 37
Sex: Female
Profession: Teacher

◆ Symptoms: When Claire came to me she was on sick leave. She suffered from tension headaches and stiffness in the neck and shoulders. She felt edgy and had totally lost her self-confidence. She had been prescribed painkillers.
◆ After the first treatment: She told me that her headache had gone and that she felt calmer and a bit spaced out.
◆ After subsequent treatments: After six treatments, she told me that her tension headache had not returned. Her neck and shoulder area was really mobile. Her friends had remarked that she looked much happier and more confident. Claire felt able to return to work.
◆ Further recommendations: One treatment a week for eight weeks and then to be reviewed.

## CASE HISTORY

Age: 57
Sex: Male
Profession: Job seeker

◆ Symptoms: Since being made redundant, Mike had felt stressed, tired out and depressed. He came to me complaining of extreme stiffness in his neck and shoulders and he suffered from recurring headaches. He had been prescribed anti-depressants by his GP.
◆ After the first treatment: He felt nice and relaxed, dreamy and sleepy and yet` remarked that he felt he had more energy than before.
◆ After subsequent treatments: His physical symptoms had greatly reduced, but most important from Mike's point of view was that his attitude to life and to the business of finding work had changed. He said he wished he and his bosses had used Indian head massage as a form of stress-management in his previous job.
◆ Further recommendations: On-going sessions whenever he felt able to come.

'It's not what you eat, but what's eating you.' Proverb

## CASE HISTORY

Age: 25
Sex: Male
Profession: Insurance Salesman

◆ Symptoms: Difficulty in expressing himself. Sleep deprivation four nights a week for the last three months. Started a new job and had moved away from home. Near to tears. He came to me for help.
◆ After the first treatment: James felt relaxed. When he came for the next treatment he was amazed his sleep pattern had greatly improved.
◆ After subsequent treatments: By the time James had had five treatments he was smiling, relaxed and settled and he felt re-energized. He said he was much more in touch with his feelings and saw things more clearly. Most importantly, he was sleeping more soundly.
◆ Further recommendations: To continue head massage treatments for a further two to three months.

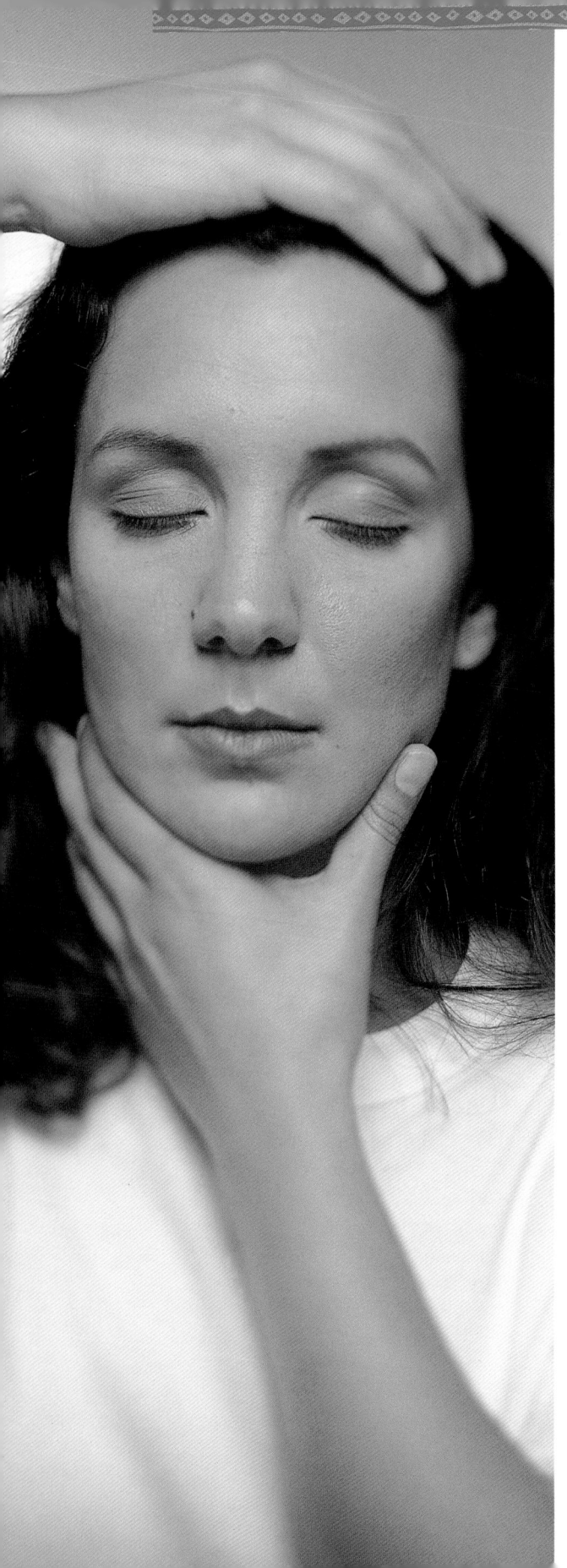

# MELT AWAY STRESS WITH INDIAN HEAD MASSAGE

Head massage is a touch therapy, which in itself creates a bond and provides comfort for my clients. Most people are starved of physical touch and may simply find human contact very therapeutic. The simple act of sitting down and being still, with someone's healing hands on your head will disperse your stress straight away. There are no language or intellectual barriers and the contact can be very valuable for anyone who is experiencing isolation or loneliness. Touch, via Indian head massage, brings about a feeling of inner peace.

Working on particular areas of the body, especially the neck and the shoulders, where stress affects major muscle groups, can bring immediate relief. Tensions are eased and fibrous knots and nodules melt away. The effeciency of the circulatory and lymphatic systems improves, toxins are dispersed from tense muscles and flexibility and fluidity of movement is restored.

As the massage proceeds, the client relaxes; his or her breathing becomes deeper and more and more oxygen is supplied to the body. It's not uncommon for a client to tell me that they have hit upon a solution to a pressing problem after experiencing an Indian head massage. The brain needs plenty of oxygenated blood! As the treatment continues, a deeper sense of relaxation is induced and I feel the client's energy level is improved. At this point some people find it helps them to open up and talk about the troubles and stresses in their lives. Many people find it easier to talk to a 'stranger' than they do to friends and relatives, who may seem too close. Talking can be very therapeutic, helping to release bottled up feelings and thoughts.

> 'If we all had half an hour of this a week, I am convinced, life would seem sunnier.'
>
> Daily Mail

Towards the end of a head massage session, my clients feel a tremendous sense of peace. The balancing of chakra energy is the icing on the cake. By releasing and freeing life force energy to flow through the client, he or she gets a boost on all levels. It is this that allows healing to take place as the client becomes connected to the wider scheme of things. A self-awareness of the qualities of love residing within the heart can be rekindled, allowing complete enjoyment of life once again. My clients always leave a treatment finding it easier to smile!

## THE END RESULT

My clients always report a lessening or disappearance of their stress-induced symptoms. They tell me that they:

- Sleep very well
- Have more energy
- Don't get headaches
- Think more clearly
- Feel good all over

By sharing the techniques in this book, you'll be able to go a long way towards getting rid of many of the physical and some of the mental symptoms of stress in your life and the lives of your partner, friends and work colleagues. Try Indian head massage and experience the difference! Or for a total physical, mental and emotional lift and a subtle balancing of the chakra energy treat yourself to a Champissage session with a qualified therapist. If you cannot find the time to go to a qualified therapist or give yourself a head massage, you might like to try some exercise in the office.

# WHAT ELSE CAN YOU DO?

Some people seem to be natural 'copers': they sail through situations that most of us would find extremely stressful with no apparent ill-effects. How do they manage it? Studies have shown that such people tend to posses certain characteristics, some of them physical and some of them mental, that help them to cope with what life throws at them. Even if we are not naturally blessed with these characteristics, most of them are things we can all cultivate if we try hard enough.

- A sense of purpose in life
- A positive outlook
- Outlets for creative self-expression
- Physical, mental and emotional fitness
- A low resting heart rate
- Physical stamina
- A good bodyweight ratio (slim but not underweight)
- An ability to express emotions (including anger) assertively
- An ability to relax thoroughly in any situation
- A sense of self worth
- A pride in your achievements
- The skills to manage your relationships so that support and enjoyment are maximized
- The ability to manage your stress in a good-humoured and flexible way

Indian head massage is guaranteed to lift you out of the hustle and bustle of everyday stress, but there are some extra things you can do to help your body to cope with the strains it has to face. The following techniques are all useful ways of dealing with stress.

- Stick to a diet low in caffeine, salt, sugar and alcohol
- Relaxation exercises
- Meditation
- Yoga
- Tai chi
- Breathing exercises
- Healthy eating
- Body massage
- Take regular breaks
- If you smoke, give up
- Learn time management
- Use relaxing herbal and essential oil baths
- Make sure that you sleep soundly
- Undertake assertiveness training
- Have a hearty laugh at least once a day

## CASE HISTORY

Age 26
Sex: Female
Profession: TV executive

◆ Symptoms: Recurring nightmares had made bedtime a misery for Sue. Her doctor had prescribed sleeping tablets but the nightmares continued. She was constantly waking up in the middle of the night, covered in sweat. She had terrible pain in her neck and shoulders and complained of a feeling of pins and needles in her upper body. Her hectic life in the fast lane had left her worn out and anxious.

◆ After the first treatment: During Indian head massage, her neck and shoulder tension eased up. Afterwards, Sue told me that it had felt like she'd been sinking into a large bowl of chocolate mousse! When she next visited me, she reported that the pain had gone completely on the day following her first treatment.

◆ After subsequent treatments: Her nightmares ceased after five treatments and she started to sleep much more soundly. Her neck and shoulder pains went completely and have not returned. Sue has much more mobility in her upper body and thanks to improved concentration, she feels much more comfortable at work. After stopping Indian head massage, she's only had a couple of bad dreams.

◆ Further recommendations: To have a head massage as often as her schedule would allow.

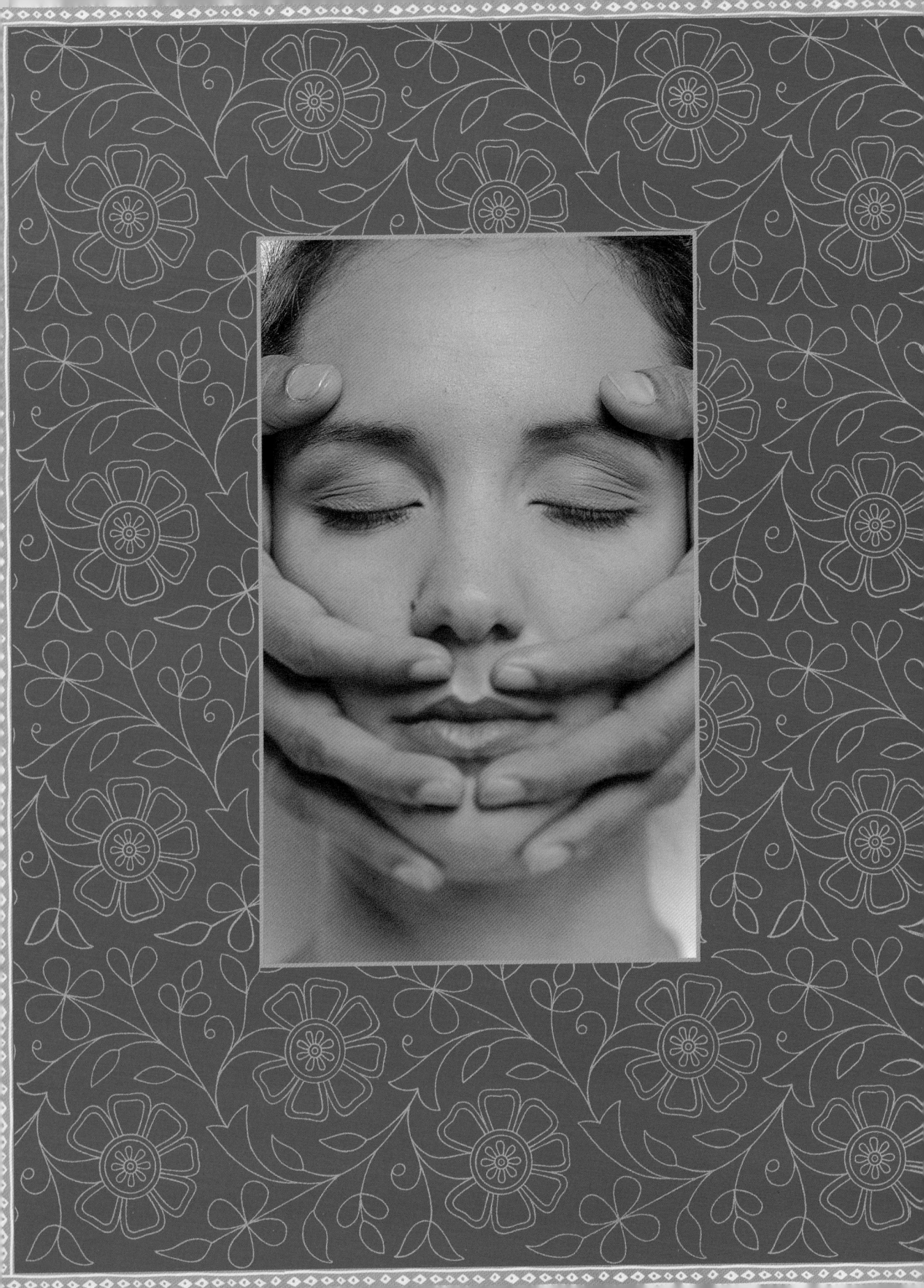

# CHAPTER 3

# Basic Massage Techniques

This chapter gives you inside information on how to prepare for and carry out Indian head massage on friends and family, with step-by-step instructions for all the techniques. You will also learn a bit about the muscles and bones inside your body so you know what the effect of your massage will be deep down.

# FIRST THINGS FIRST

◆ You do not need to use any oils or cream.

◆ Ask the person who is receiving the massage to remove any neck-chains or earrings. If they want to remove their shoes they can do so.

◆ Ask them to sit down in an upright chair where you will feel comfortable massaging them without having to tense your own arms and shoulders.

◆ When they are seated, make sure they do not have their knees crossed or their feet crossed at the ankles.

◆ Ask them to place the soles of their feet firmly on the ground and place their hands in their lap.

◆ Stand behind them.

# GET CONNECTED

◆ Lay your hands very lightly on the top of the other person's head.

◆ Relax. Now ask the other person to relax and do the following breathing exercise with you.

◆ Close your mouth and breathe in and out, deeply and gently, three times through your nostrils.

Both of you will become more grounded and in touch if you use this simple technique before every massage. It relaxes you and stills your mind, concentrating your energy on the task in hand.

## 'When the breath is steady, ... so is the mind ...' Hatha Yoga Pradipika

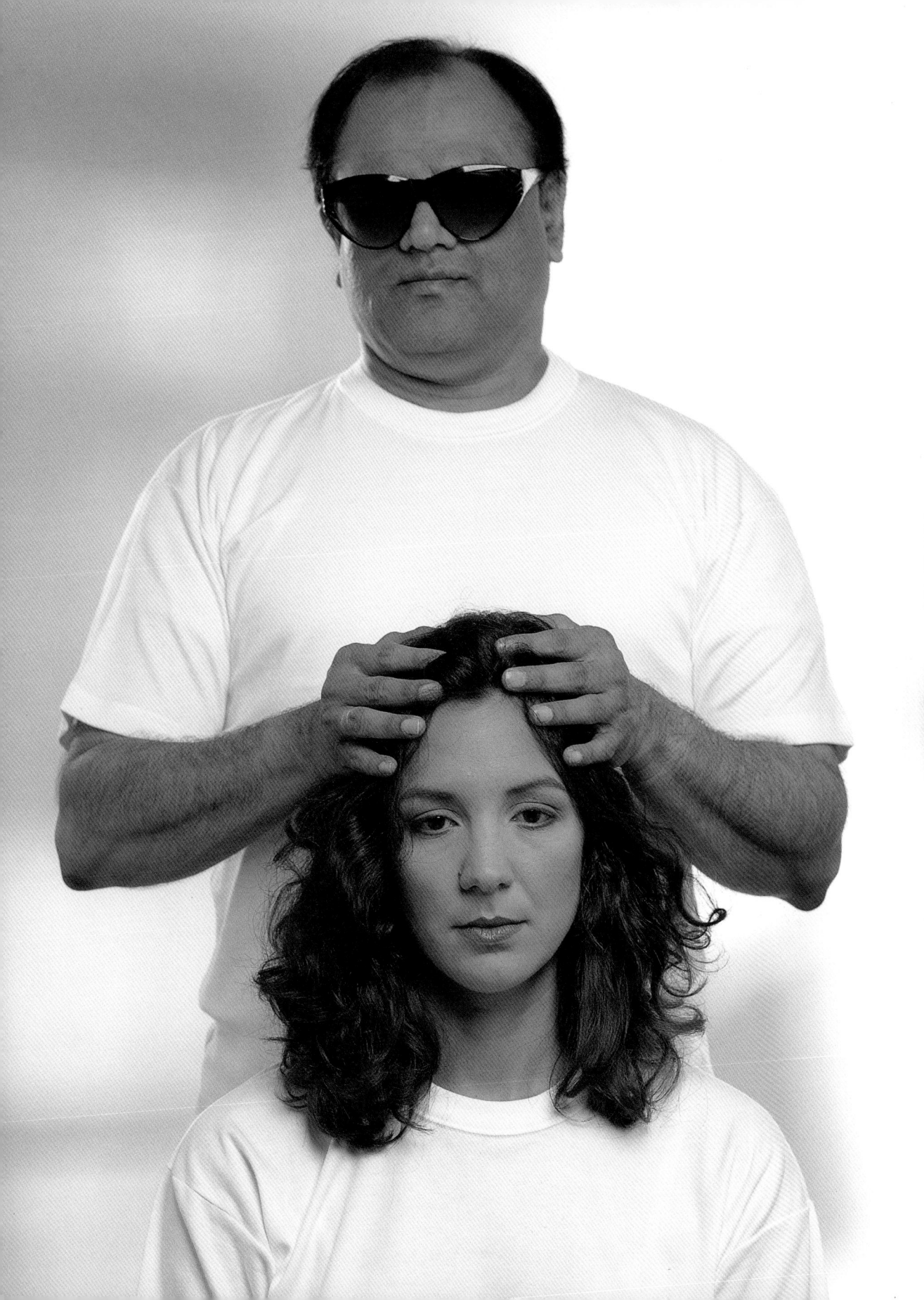

# FRICTION OR A RUB?

Throughout the following chapter, and the chapters on 'Partners and Lovers' and 'Self Massage', you will find movements described as 'friction' or 'rubbing': so what's the difference? Friction requires fairly heavy pressure and should cause the skin to move over the bones of the scalp with your hand. A rub is a lighter motion: your hand should move over the surface of the skin.

# YOUR SHOULDERS

Most people find that one of the first places they experience tension is in their shoulders. The shoulders are designed for total flexibility and possess a wider range of movements than any other joint in the body. However, if you sit for long periods in front of your computer screen or slouch your way around your office and home, you force the muscles in your shoulders to do far more work than they were ever designed to. You may find that your shoulders slowly stiffen up and lose mobility. As well as being painful in itself, this has an immediate effect on the rest of the body, restricting the ribs and how deeply you breathe, slowing down the circulation, creating headaches and impeding digestion, as well as affecting posture and throwing the whole body out of balance. Massaging this region can relieve the tension in the overworked muscles and release trapped energy.

The more responsibilities we have – be they from work, running a home, looking after a family or just generally sorting our lives out – the more likely it is that we'll begin to feel that 'burdened' feeling which often translates into a state of tension in the shoulders. The expression 'to shoulder responsibility' is not just a throwaway phrase. It actually reflects a physical reality, which can really weigh us down and often feel oppressive.

Most people continually carry their shoulders in a raised position, which creates a tremendous amount of tension in the whole of the upper back, as the shoulders, rather than just hanging as nature intended, have to fight against the force of gravity to remain constantly raised. Massage can help to relieve the stress that causes us to tense up in the first place as well as loosening the whole shoulder area and bringing your shoulders down to where they should be.

The shoulders are a very accurate barometer of our ability to flow and express ourselves freely. If your shoulders have slowly become tight and immobile over the years, then perhaps you are also in danger of losing your sense of spontaneity and adventure. Releasing the tension in your shoulders can also release an ability to express your ambitions and feelings freely, allowing you to plunge into life, rather than tiptoeing around the edges.

Next time you are undressed, stand in front of a mirror and have a look at your shoulders. You may be surprised to notice how unbalanced your body has become: you may see that one shoulder is held higher than the other or that both shoulders seem to be almost touching your ears.

# Bones of the Shoulder

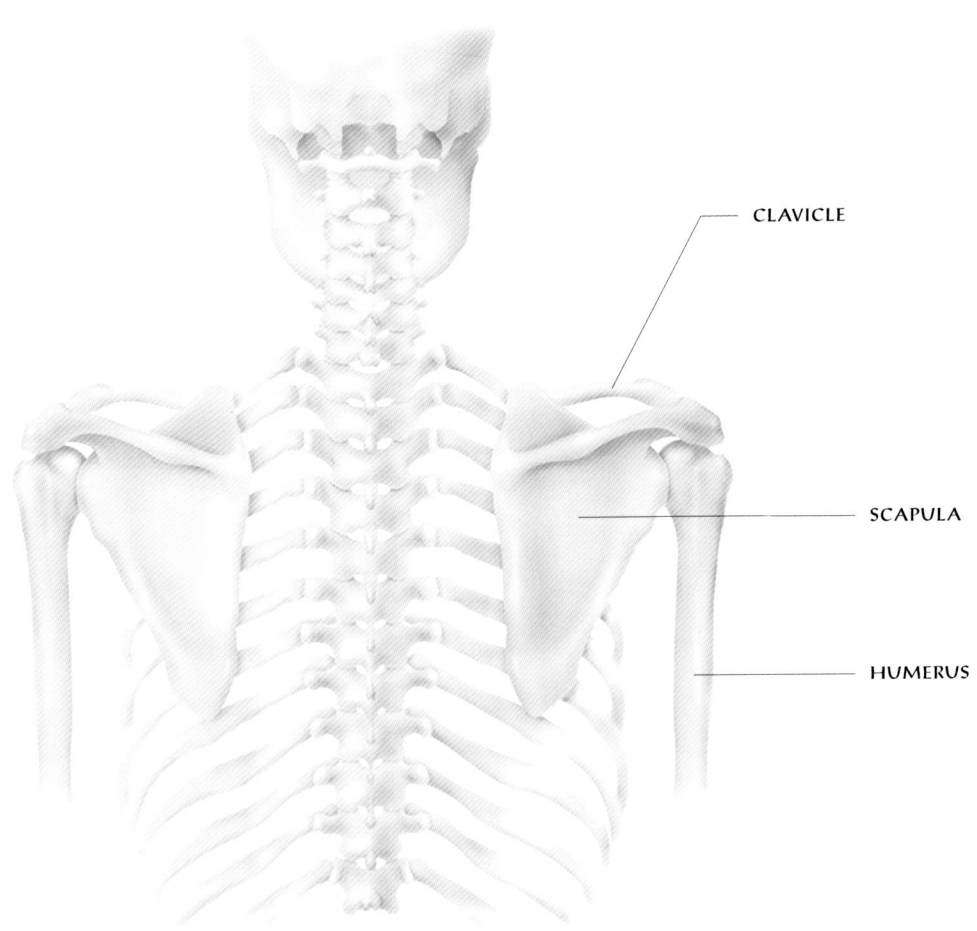

CLAVICLE

SCAPULA

HUMERUS

# Muscles of the Shoulder

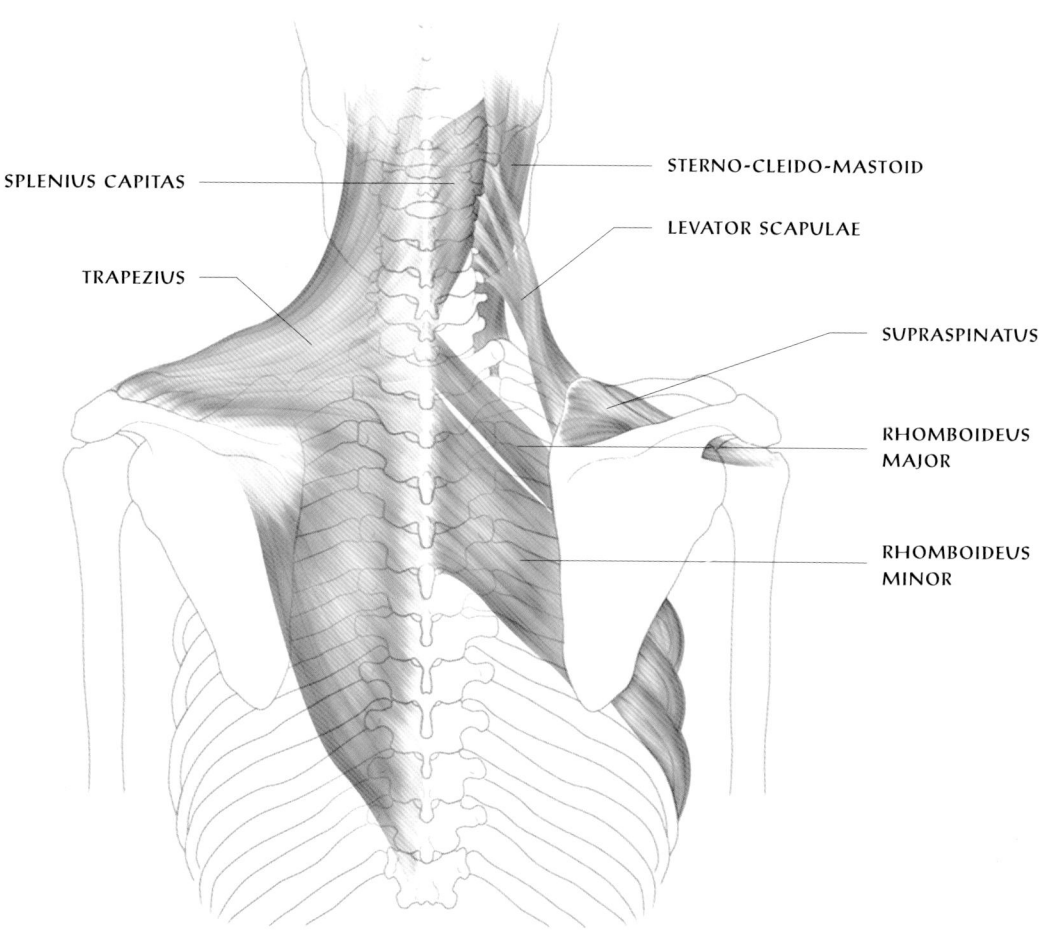

SPLENIUS CAPITAS

STERNO-CLEIDO-MASTOID

LEVATOR SCAPULAE

TRAPEZIUS

SUPRASPINATUS

RHOMBOIDEUS MAJOR

RHOMBOIDEUS MINOR

# SHOULDER MASSAGE

### THUMB PUSH

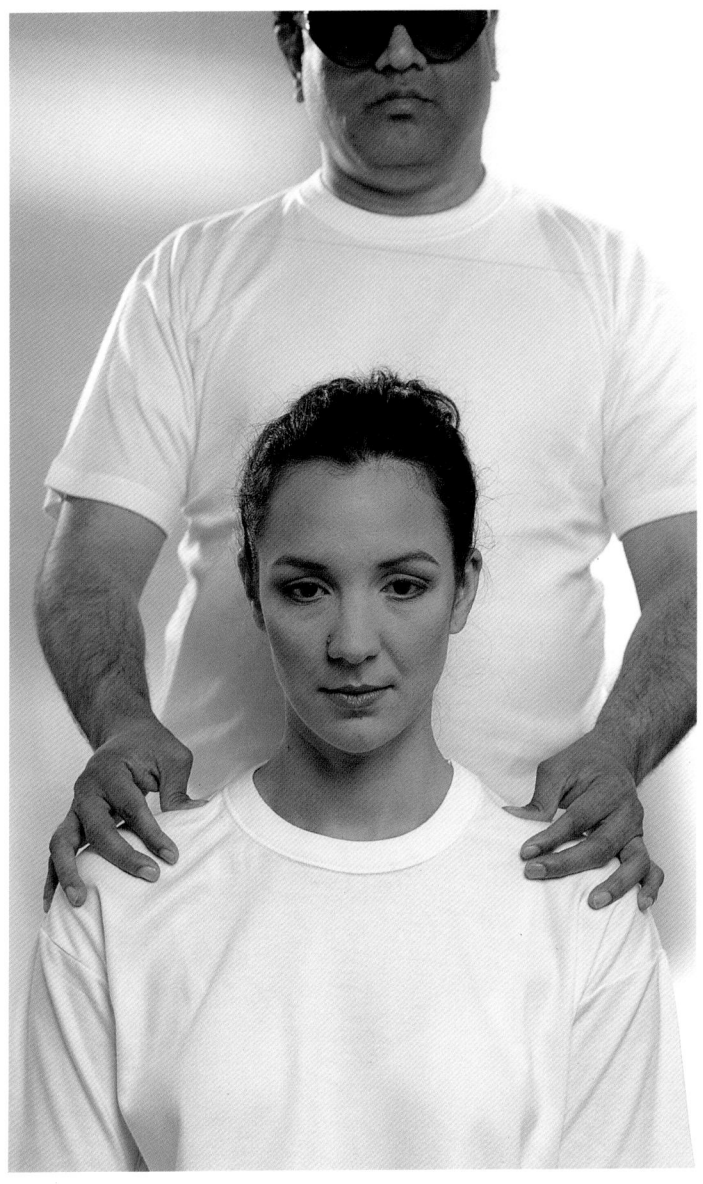

◆ Place the palms of your hands at the corners of the shoulders with thumbs resting above the shoulder blades. Push with your thumbs, using medium pressure, up and over the shoulder muscles. Now pull back the muscles, dragging your fingers towards your thumbs, using medium pressure. Repeat the action at the middle of the shoulders, then again at the junction of the neck and shoulders.

◆ By applying pressure on the shoulder muscles, you are helping to break down knots and nodules.

In effect, you are squeezing out toxins and softening up the muscles.

'[Head massage] works to promote physical and psychological well-being.' Elle Magazine

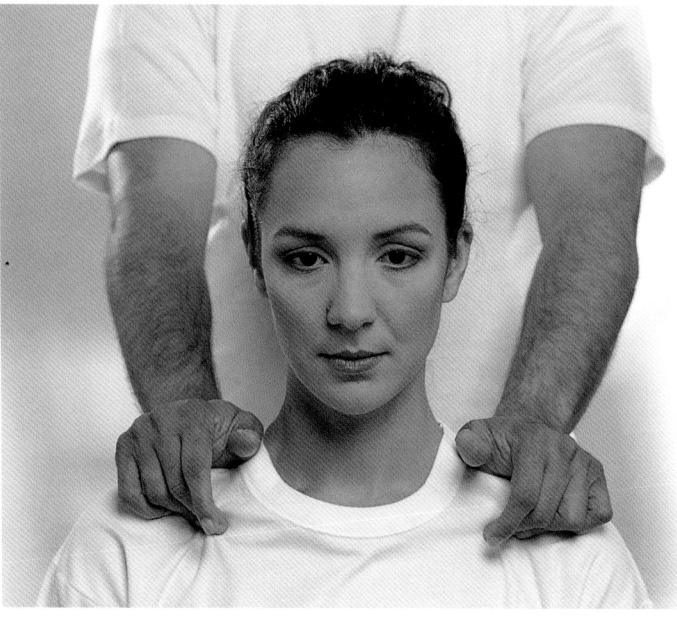

## HEEL PUSH

◆ In some cases, you may not be able to do the thumb push because the shoulders are too broad. In this case, you can use the heels of your hands instead of your thumbs. This allows you to exert more pressure while you work the same area without becoming tired.

◆ By applying pressure on the shoulder muscles, you are helping to break down knots and nodules. In effect, you are squeezing out toxins and softening up the muscles.

## FINGER PULLS

◆ Place your thumbs between the shoulder blades and your fingers near the neck in front of the shoulder muscles. Pull back the muscles, dragging your fingers towards your thumbs, using medium pressure. Repeat at the middle of the shoulders, and again further along the muscle near the corner of the shoulders.

◆ By applying pressure on the shoulder muscles, you are helping to break down knots and nodules. In effect, you are squeezing out toxins and softening up the muscles.

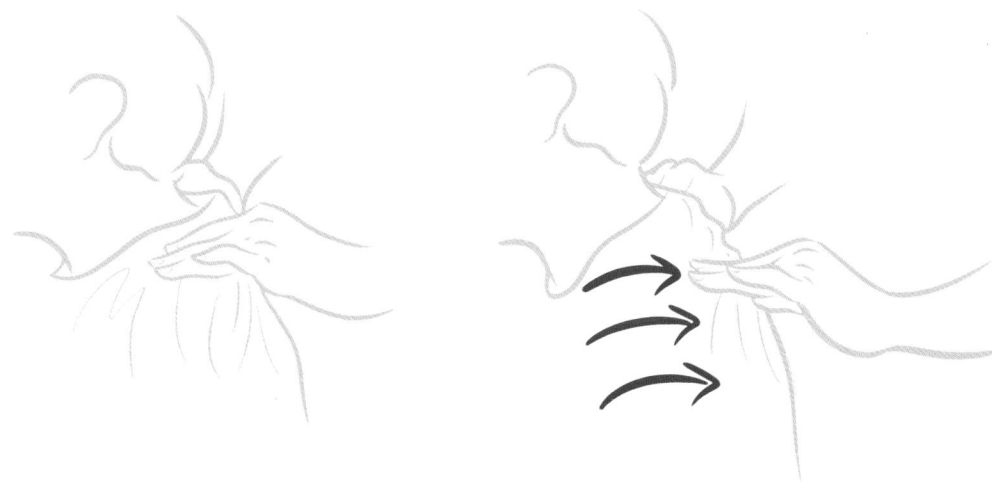

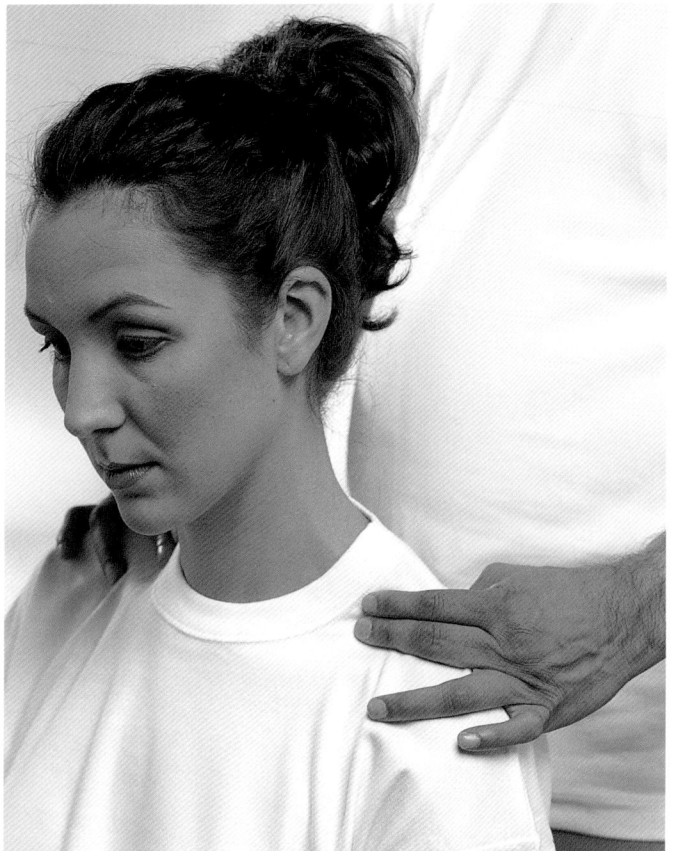

## PICK UP AND SQUEEZE

◆ Place the palms of your hands on the corners of the shoulders with your thumbs behind the shoulder muscles and fingers in front. Push your thumbs towards your fingers gathering as much muscle as possible. Squeeze using medium pressure and hold for a few seconds, then let go. Repeat at the middle of the shoulders. Repeat near the neck.

◆ This technique helps to squeeze out toxins from the tight muscles, making them softer and more mobile. It also helps to break down fibrous adhesions.

'The beauty of this technique is that you don't have to undress to be treated. Consequently, you can practise your new found skill on anyone at any time.' Here's Health

## CHAMPI

◆ Place your hands together in a prayer position, keeping your wrists relaxed. Make quick, light hitting movements with your little fingers across the shoulders – touching the muscles only.
◆ This will stimulate the blood circulation.

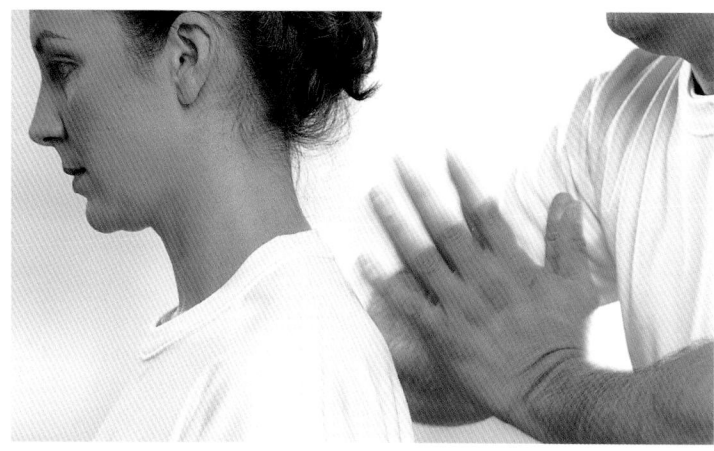

## IRONING DOWN

◆ Place the heels of your hands on either side of the neck. Point your fingers towards the corners of the shoulders. Apply medium pressure and slide both hands across the shoulder muscles to the edge of the shoulder.
◆ This helps to drain away toxins and bring the shoulders down, and is a superb muscle relaxer.

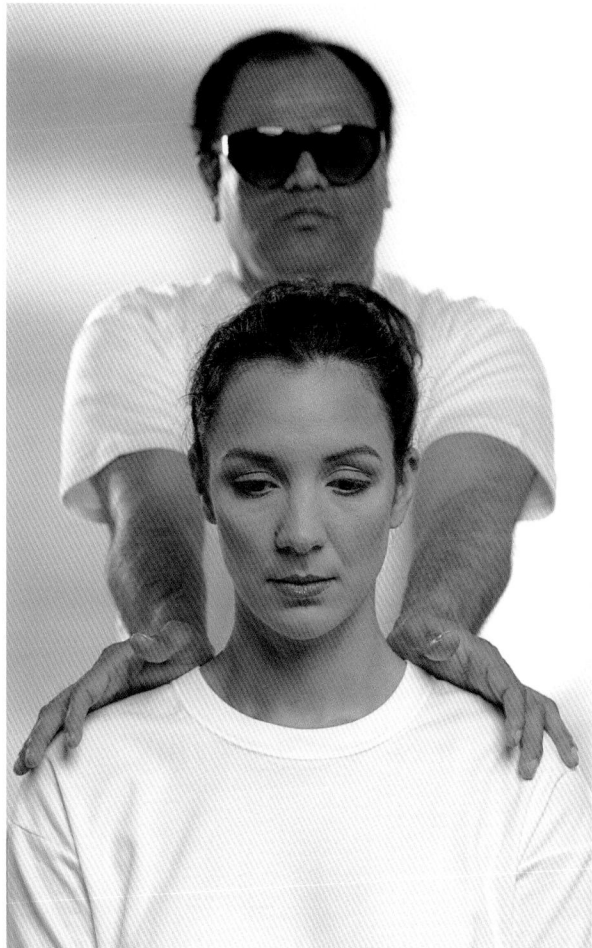

# YOUR UPPER ARMS

The upper arms are components of the shoulder girdle and so there is a direct relationship between the arms and the shoulders. The main muscles of the upper arm have their origins in the shoulder blades, and tension in the shoulders can spread to the upper arm if untreated. In the same way tension in the upper arms can spread to the shoulders if untreated. Tension can creep into your arms due to working long hours on a computer or

## Bones of the Upper Arm

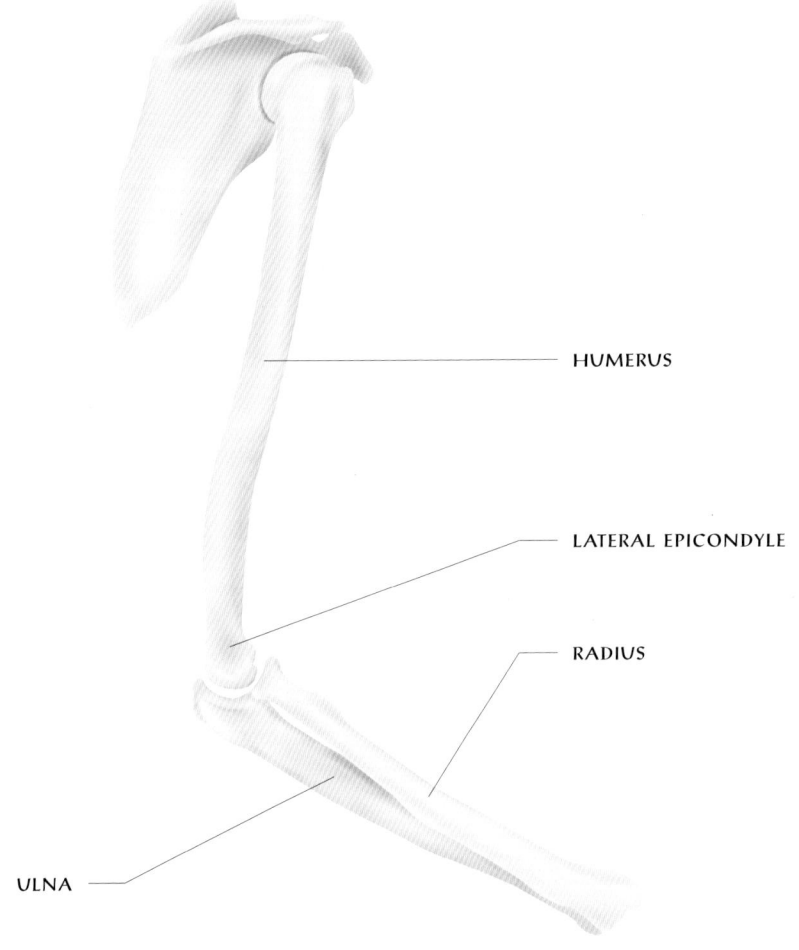

HUMERUS

LATERAL EPICONDYLE

RADIUS

ULNA

constantly carrying a heavy bag. If you cannot avoid long hours at a computer, make sure your work station is as ergonomically sound as possible and take short, frequent breaks, stretching your neck and arms as often as possible (see 'Office Exercises' page 24).

Because of the integral relationship between your head, neck, shoulders and upper arms, it is important to treat all of these areas during a head massage.

## Muscles of the Upper Arm

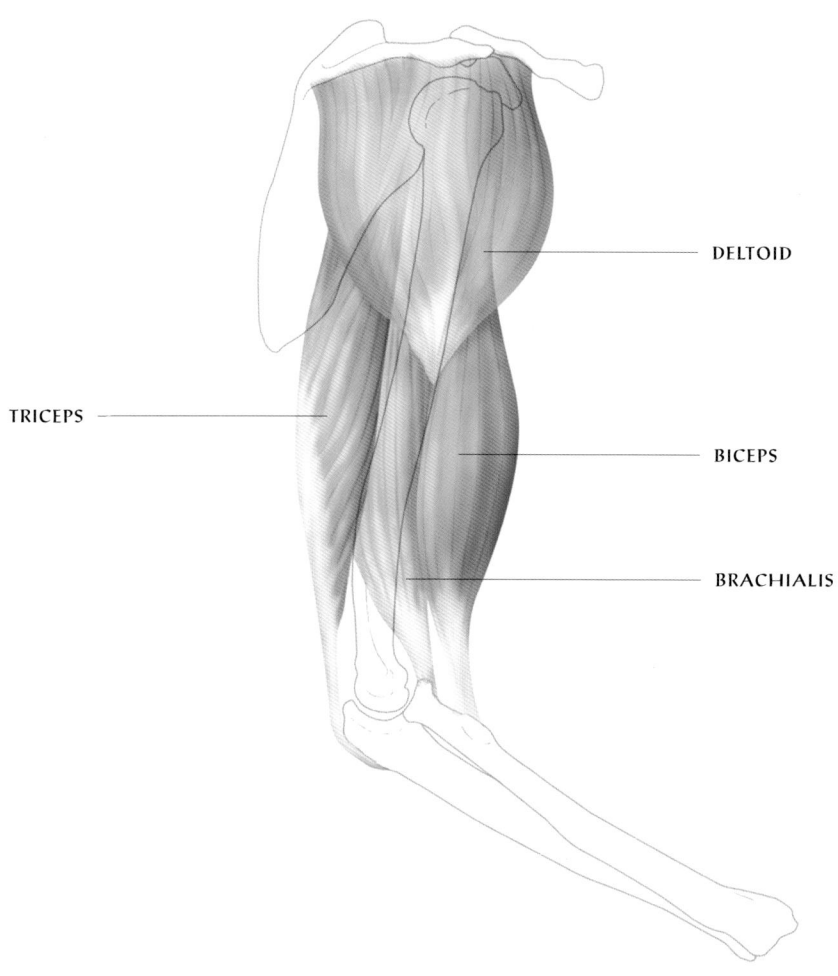

DELTOID

TRICEPS

BICEPS

BRACHIALIS

# UPPER ARM MASSAGE

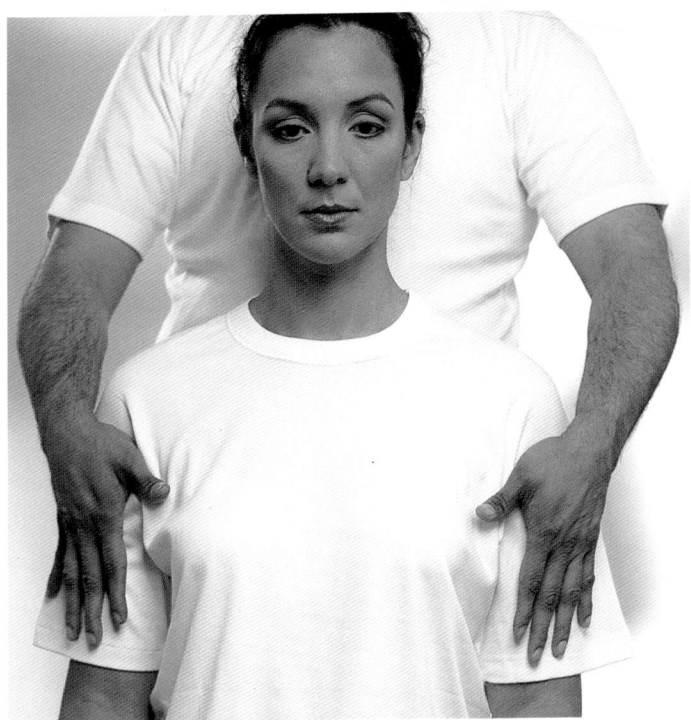

### IRONING DOWN

◆ Ironing down the shoulders leads naturally on to working with the upper arms: continue the movement with the heels of your hands to relax and loosen the arm muscles. Work from the top of the arm down to the elbow, using firm pressure. Go down the sides of the arms, and then down the front of the arms.

◆ Remember to repeat these techniques three times for maximum benefit.

'There is but one temple in the universe, and that is the body of man. Nothing is holier than that high form.' Novalis

### SKIN BOOST

Massage helps to drain away the toxins that gather in your skin and muscles, and it improves your circulation. Regular massage sessions can help to improve the texture and the tone of your skin, leaving it noticeably silkier and smoother.

'The sense of relaxation and well-being that head massage brings helps considerably to counteract the many stresses and strains of modern living.' Yoga and Health

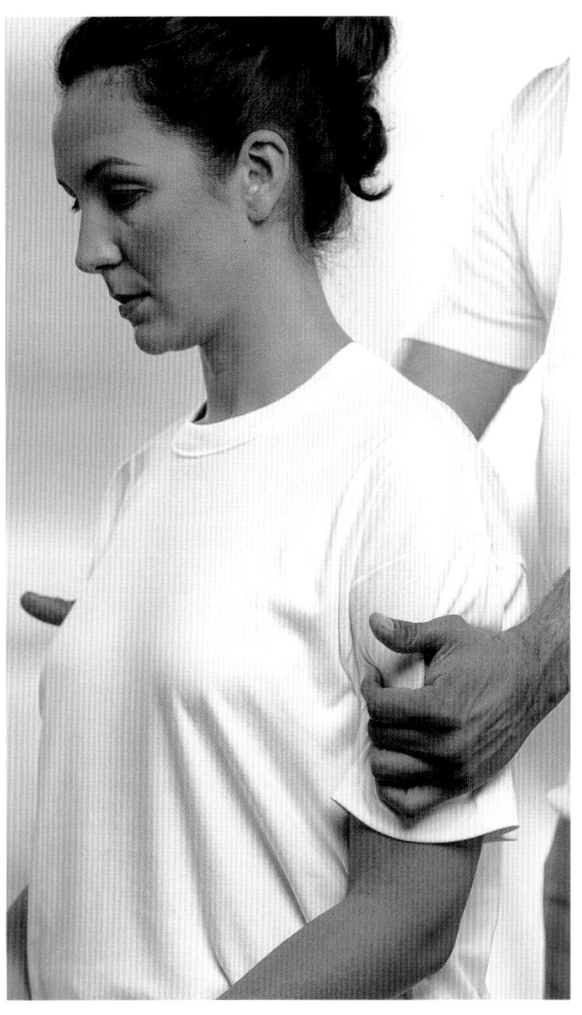

### HEEL ROLL

◆ Place your hands on top of the arms (on the deltoid muscles), fingers in front, heels behind. With firm pressure, roll the heels of your hands forwards over the muscles to arrive at your fingertips. Repeat at the middle of the upper arm, then again just above the elbow. Repeat the whole process twice more.

◆ Make sure that you do not pinch the muscles at the end of the stroke and spoil the effect!

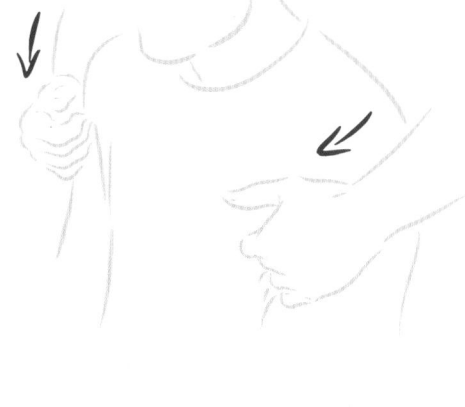

# Your Neck

The neck is a complex region containing an elaborate lattice of muscles and neck vertebrae which allow the head to move in a variety of directions. Most of the important arteries, veins and nerves pass through the neck. No wonder it gets tense so often!

In its normal state, the head is designed to balance perfectly upon the neck vertebrae without imposing any strain. However, because many of us stick our chins forward a little when we are talking, concentrating or watching television, our heads are thrown out of alignment. This results in the neck muscles tensing up to take the full weight of the head, and a vicious circle is created. The neck muscles are constantly compensating for an unbalanced head and end up permanently contracted. This causes tremendous congestion

## Bones of the Neck

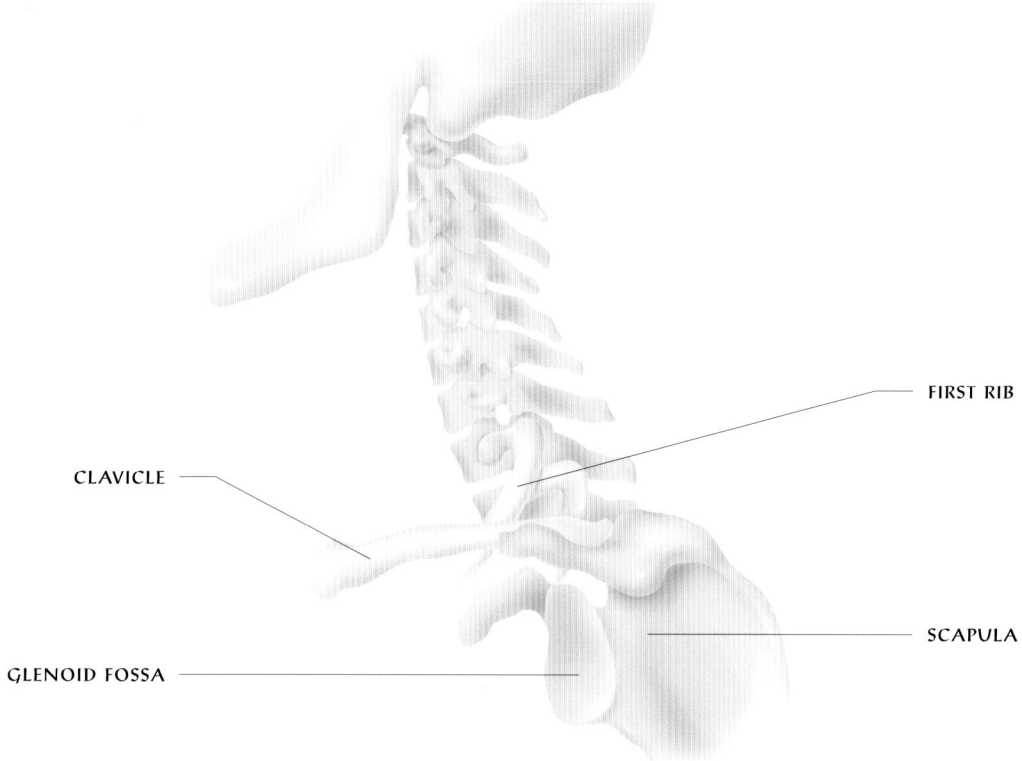

FIRST RIB

CLAVICLE

SCAPULA

GLENOID FOSSA

and tightness, reduces neck mobility, and often results in tension headaches, migraines and eyestrain. In addition, if the neck becomes tight and stiff, it can have a knock-on effect on the shoulders. The neck also comes under pressure if we habitually tilt our heads to one side. This can lead to one set of neck muscles becoming overconstricted, while the opposite set become weakened, resulting in neckache and even in the neck vertebrae becoming displaced.

The neck is designed to be highly mobile. However, as we get older, our neck muscles almost inevitably become tense and stiff, and it becomes more difficult to move our head freely. Since the neck and throat region is normally associated with communication, stiffness or restriction here can affect our ability to express ourselves freely and spontaneously.

## Muscles of the Neck

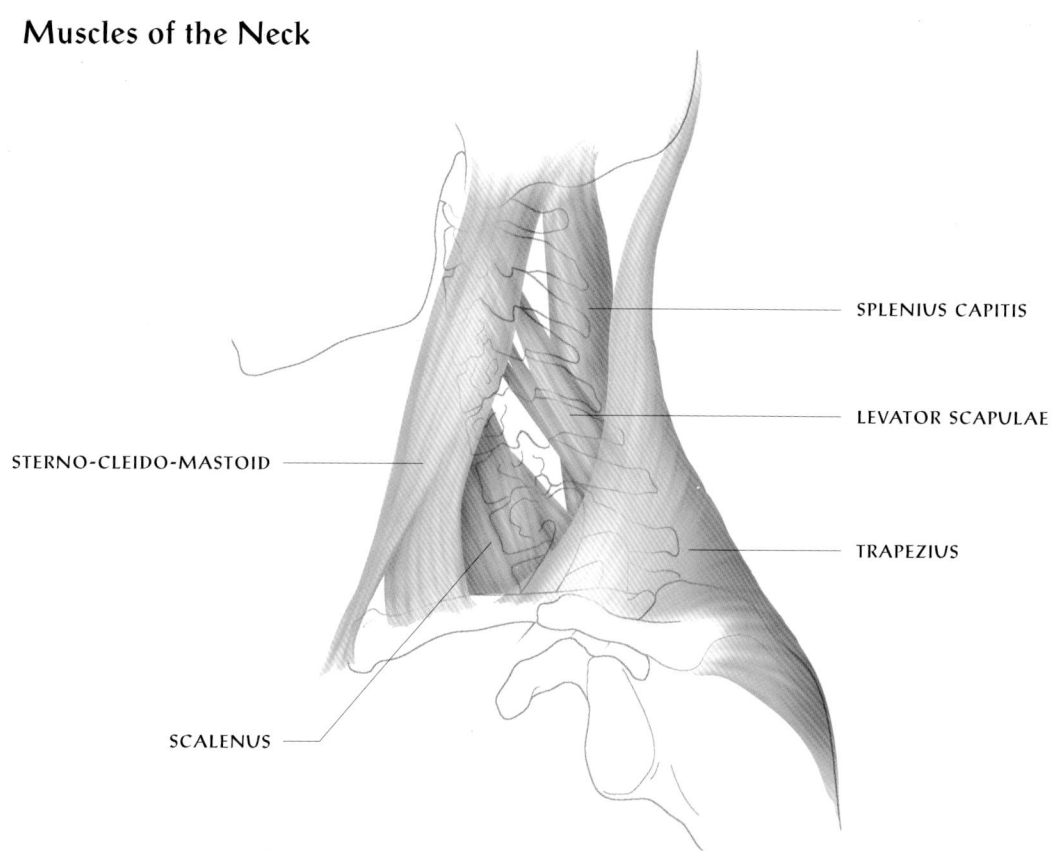

SPLENIUS CAPITIS

LEVATOR SCAPULAE

STERNO-CLEIDO-MASTOID

TRAPEZIUS

SCALENUS

# NECK MASSAGE

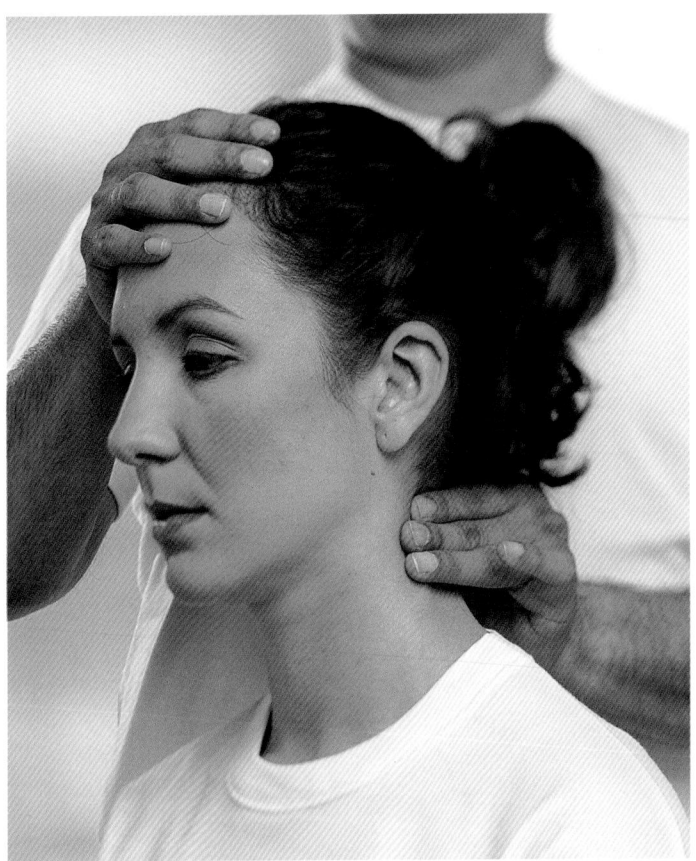

## GRASP AND PULL BACK

◆ With one hand on the forehead, tilt the neck back slightly. With the other hand, spread your thumb and fingers as far as possible on either side of the base of the neck. Using medium pressure, slide your hand up to the top of the neck, grasp the flesh and pull it back. Grasp at the middle of the neck and pull back and again at the base of the neck and pull back.

◆ This is a soft tissue mobilization technique that loosens up the neck muscles.

## NECK BEAUTY

The neck is one of the most sensual parts of a woman's body. It is also one of the first to show signs of ageing. To keep your neck supple and young-looking moisurize it well every day and carry out the neck exercises on page 119 in addition to the neck massage techniques shown here.

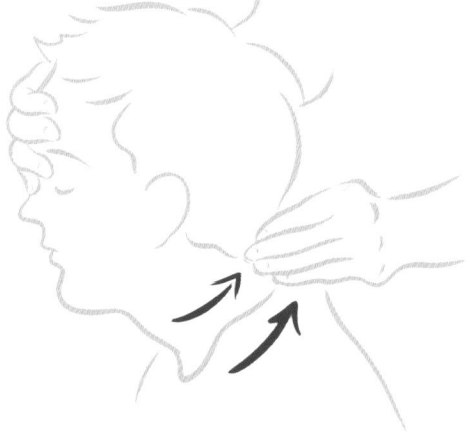

*'...incredibly sensitive fingers can alternately soothe and stimulate the head, neck, shoulders and even the ears, resulting in a feeling of lightness...'* Options

## NECK TIPS

• Choose a pillow that supports your neck well.

• Avoid lying on your front: turning your head to one side to breathe will strain your neck muscles.

• If you work at a computer, adjust the height of your monitor so you can look straight at it without tilting your head.

## FRICTION UNDER THE OCCIPUT

◆ Next, warm up the muscles underneath the occiput by using your fingertips to create gentle friction at the base of the skull. Support the forehead and work your way back and forth from behind the ear to the top of the spine. Repeat this on the other side of the head.

◆ The attachments of many muscles are located here. These very often become tight and congested and can begin to generate headaches. This technique helps to loosen up congested muscles and releases toxins to be drained away.

## HEEL RUB UNDER THE OCCIPUT

◆ Place your right hand over the front of the forehead to support the head, then tilt the head forwards just slightly. Place the heel of you left hand against the base of the skull and rub lightly and briskly over the surface of the skin.

◆ This stimulates the blood and lymphatic circulation and drains toxins away. It is an excellent technique for relieving the pain of strained muscles in the neck.

# A touch can melt away your tension ...

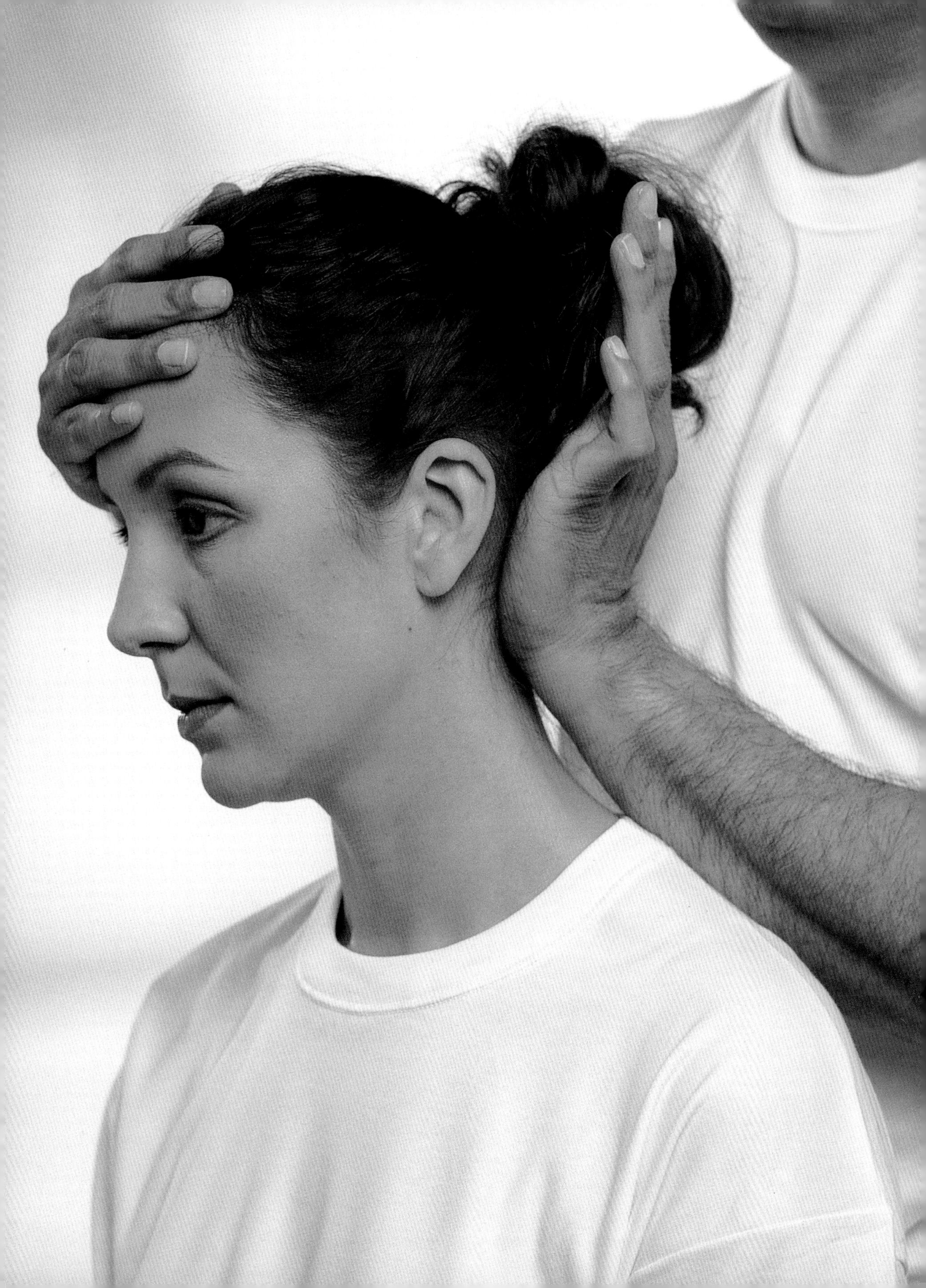

# YOUR SCALP

When we are troubled or making an effort to concentrate, we instinctively frown, causing our forehead and temples to become tense and congested. Indeed, over time, frowning in this way causes permanent lines and wrinkles. Furthermore, if the muscles around the temples become tight, this constricts the flow of blood around the head, leading to headaches and eyestrain, and possibly contributing to the hair turning grey around the

## Bones of the Scalp

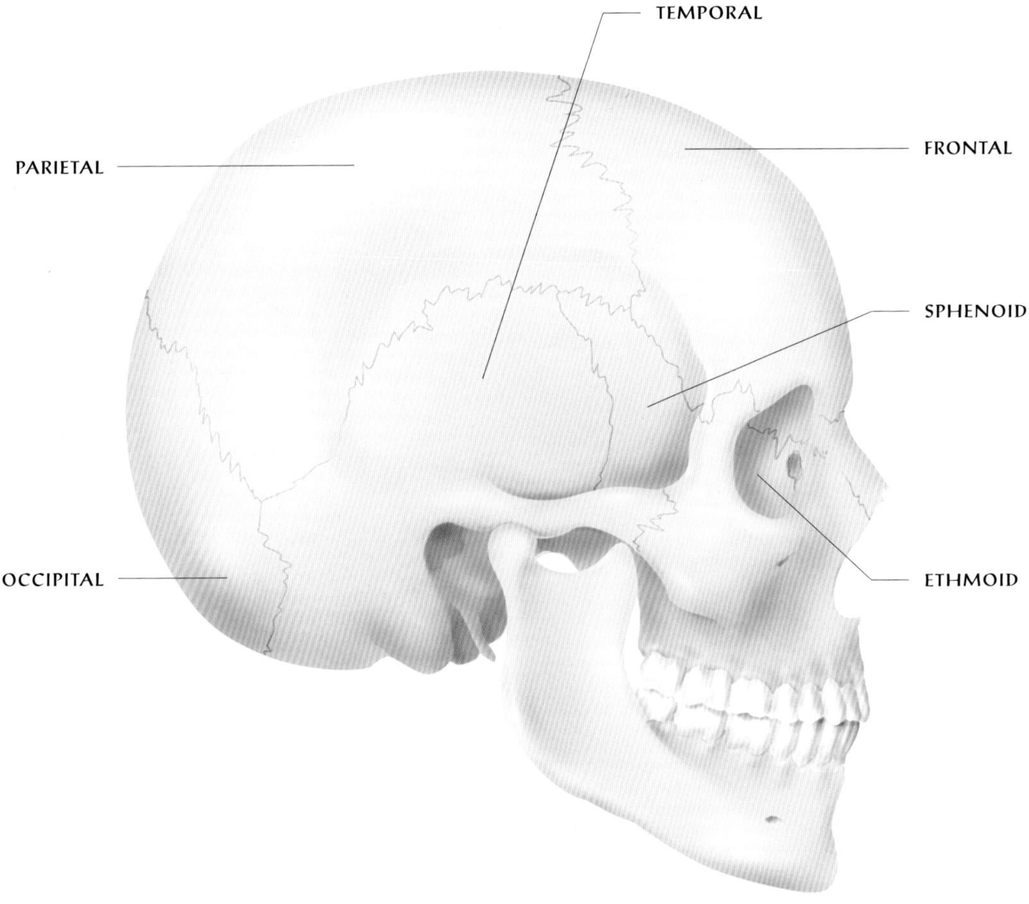

TEMPORAL

FRONTAL

PARIETAL

SPHENOID

OCCIPITAL

ETHMOID

temples as the hair roots are slowly starved of nutrients. You can tell how tense the scalp muscles are when you try a friction movement: the skin on the scalp should move freely over the bone. The tenser the muscles, the tighter the skin will feel and the less it will move. Loosening the tense muscles restores the flow of blood, improving concentration and boosting the health of your hair.

## Muscles of the Scalp

INTERMEDIATE TENDON

FRONTALIS

OCCIPITALIS

TEMPORALIS

# SCALP MASSAGE

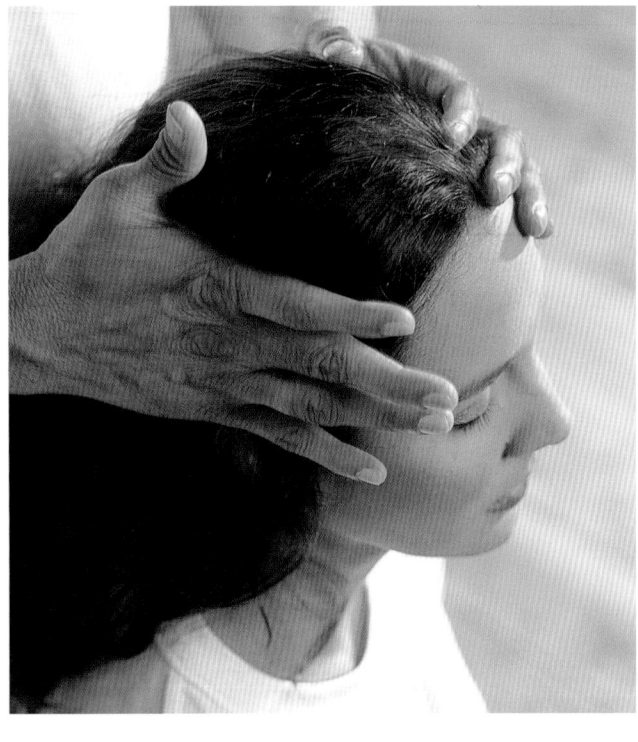

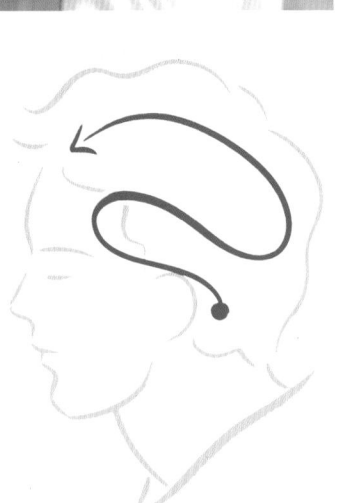

## WINDSCREEN WIPER

◆ Place your hand in front of the ear with your fingers on the forehead to support the head. Following the given route, use the ball of the other hand to carry out a light rubbing movement over the other side of the head. Repeat this on the opposite side of the head, then repeat twice more on both sides.

◆ This movement is designed to warm up and stimulate the scalp, improving the overall circulation.

## NATURAL PROTECTION

Massaging the head helps to spread the natural oils produced by the scalp along the whole length of the hair, allowing it to protect and condition right to the tips.

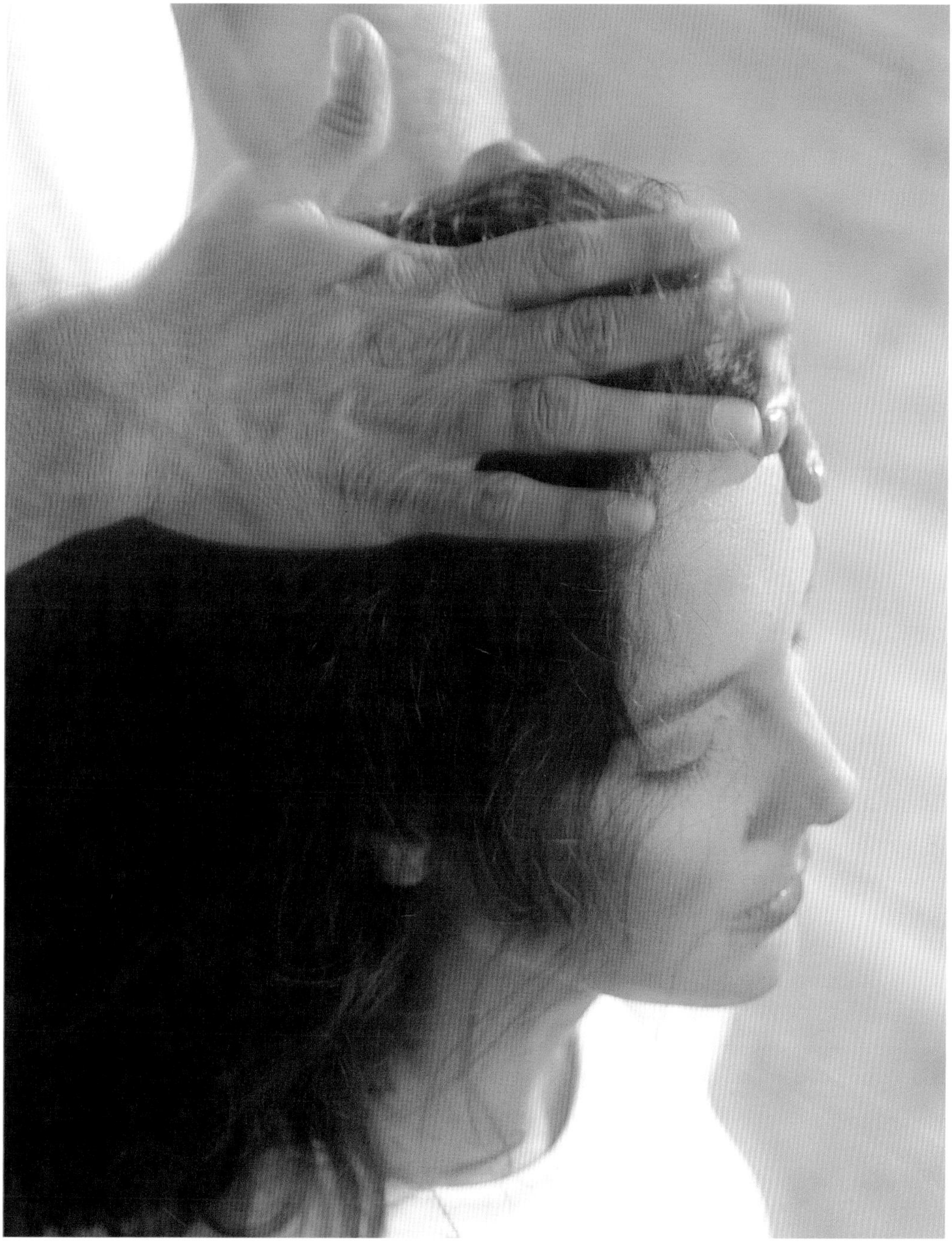

## HEALTHY SCALP – HEALTHY HAIR

Massaging the scalp improves the circulation, helping to nourish the hair from the roots and drain away any toxins that may accumulate. A regular massage will keep your scalp in tip top condition and help your hair to feel thicker and shinier.

### WHOLE HAND FRICTION

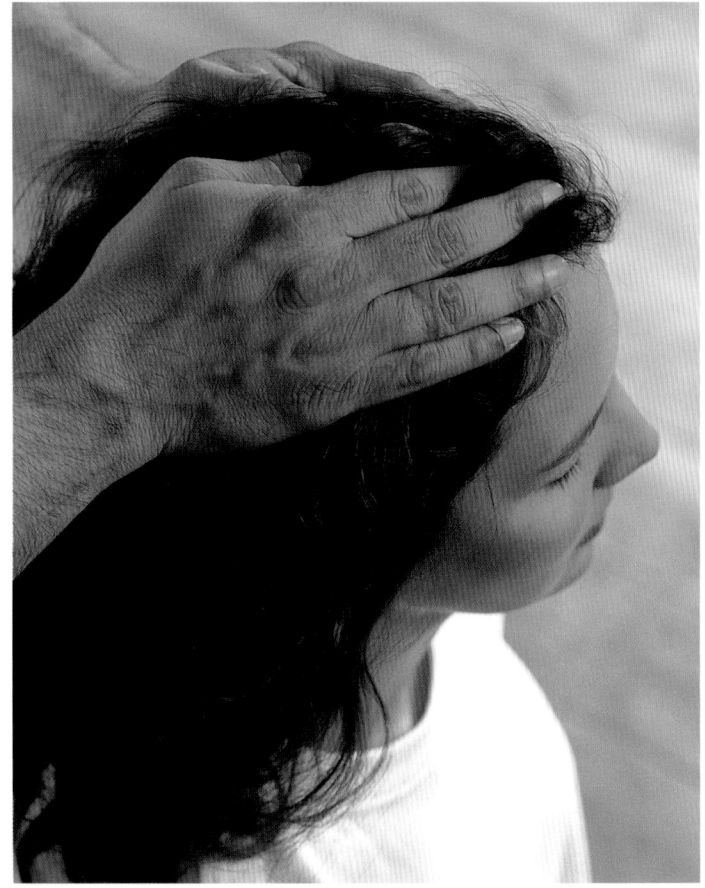

◆ This is a friction movement and not a rub. Do not allow your hands to slide over the scalp. The scalp should move under your hand.

◆ Place both hands above the ears with your fingers pointing forwards. While the head is supported by one hand, apply firm pressure with the whole of the other hand, including your fingertips and the heel. Move the scalp up and down. Move the hand to a new position slightly above the previous on. Repeat the same action. Repeat the sequence on the other side of the head.

◆ This movement loosens up the tight subcutaneous scalp muscles.

## RUFFLING

◆ Open the fingers of one hand and, keeping your wrist relaxed and supporting the head with your other hand, lightly ruffle the entire head of hair.

◆ Most people really enjoy this. The lighter the touch the better. Remember to keep your wrist loose.

### HAIR TIPS

• Shampoo strips your hair of the natural oils that protect and condition it. Try not to use shampoo more than twice a week.

• Allow your hair to dry naturally or leave it until it is almost dry before you use a hairdryer.

• Hair is especially fragile when it is wet: use a wide-toothed comb and comb it from the ends, working back to the roots.

'The ancient art of Indian head massage puts the power of stress relief at your fingertips. Expert Narendra Mehta's step-by-step technique will help you revitalise even the most sluggish spirits.' Here's Health

## PLUCKING

◆ Soft landing, quick take off!

◆ With your fingers outstretched, land softly on the head. On making contact, spring off, bringing your fingers and thumbs together. Land in a different position, with your fingers again outstretched. Repeat this energetic movement until you have covered the top of the head.

◆ This is a stimulating technique which brings the circulation to the surface.

'When energy is rebalanced, one invariably feels more alive, energized, relaxed and better able to cope with life's pressures.'

Harpers and Queen

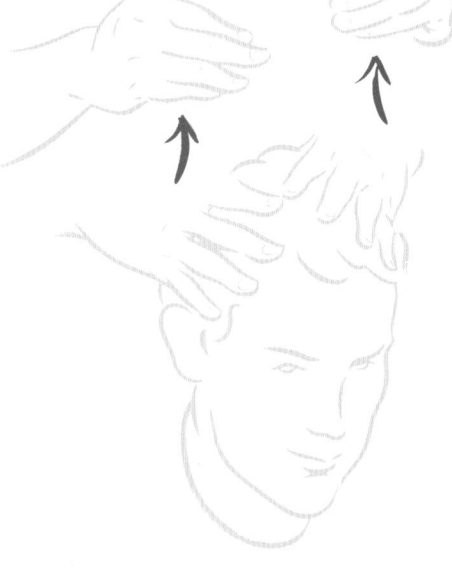

## STROKING

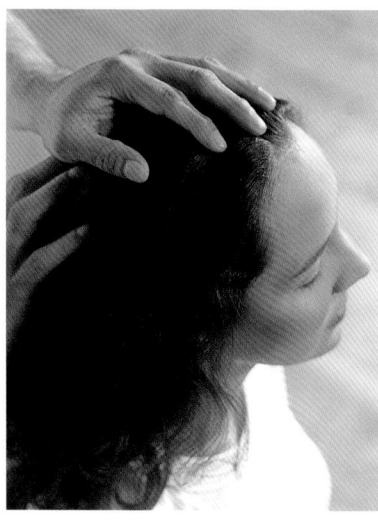

◆ By using stroking techniques you can intensify the feelings of relaxation. There are two stroking techniques:

1   Place one hand flat over the top of the head with the fingers pointing forwards at the beginning of the hairline and gently bring the hand towards the back of the head. Follow with the other hand so that a wave-like continuity is established and the person is unaware of where one stroke begins and another finishes.

2   Use a similar stroking action while running your fingers and the fingernails of both hands through the hair. Use the same wave-like movement as in 1.

◆ This will remove any feelings of stress and make the other person feel calm and nurtured.

## MAGIC TOUCH

Touch has the power to affect us on several different levels:

• It can physically relax tight muscles and so relieve pain.

• It can calm tense or troubled emotions, making us feel nurtured and cared for.

• It can be energizing as well as relaxing, leaving you feeling refreshed and uplifted.

## TABLA PLAYING

◆ Use your fingertips to gently tap on the scalp. Imagine that you are playing the piano (or the Indian tabla). Do this until you have covered the entire head.
◆ This stimulates the circulation and is surprisingly energizing.

## SQUEEZE AND LIFT (OPPOSITE PAGE)

◆ Place your fingers on top of the head with the heels of your hands behind the ears. Keep your elbows out at right angles. Squeeze inwards with your heels using medium pressure, then lift the scalp with the heels of your hands. Hold for three seconds and then let go. Repeat with the heels of the hands above the ears and then in front of the ears.
◆ This movement is excellent for releasing tension headaches.

'He who realizes the truth of the body can then come to know the truth of the universe.' Ratnasara

## RELIEVING HEADACHES

Headaches caused by tension and stress seem to be an inevitable part of modern life. Painkillers may block the 'pain messages' and relieve the pain, but massage tackles the problem at its source – relaxing the tense muscles that cause the problem.

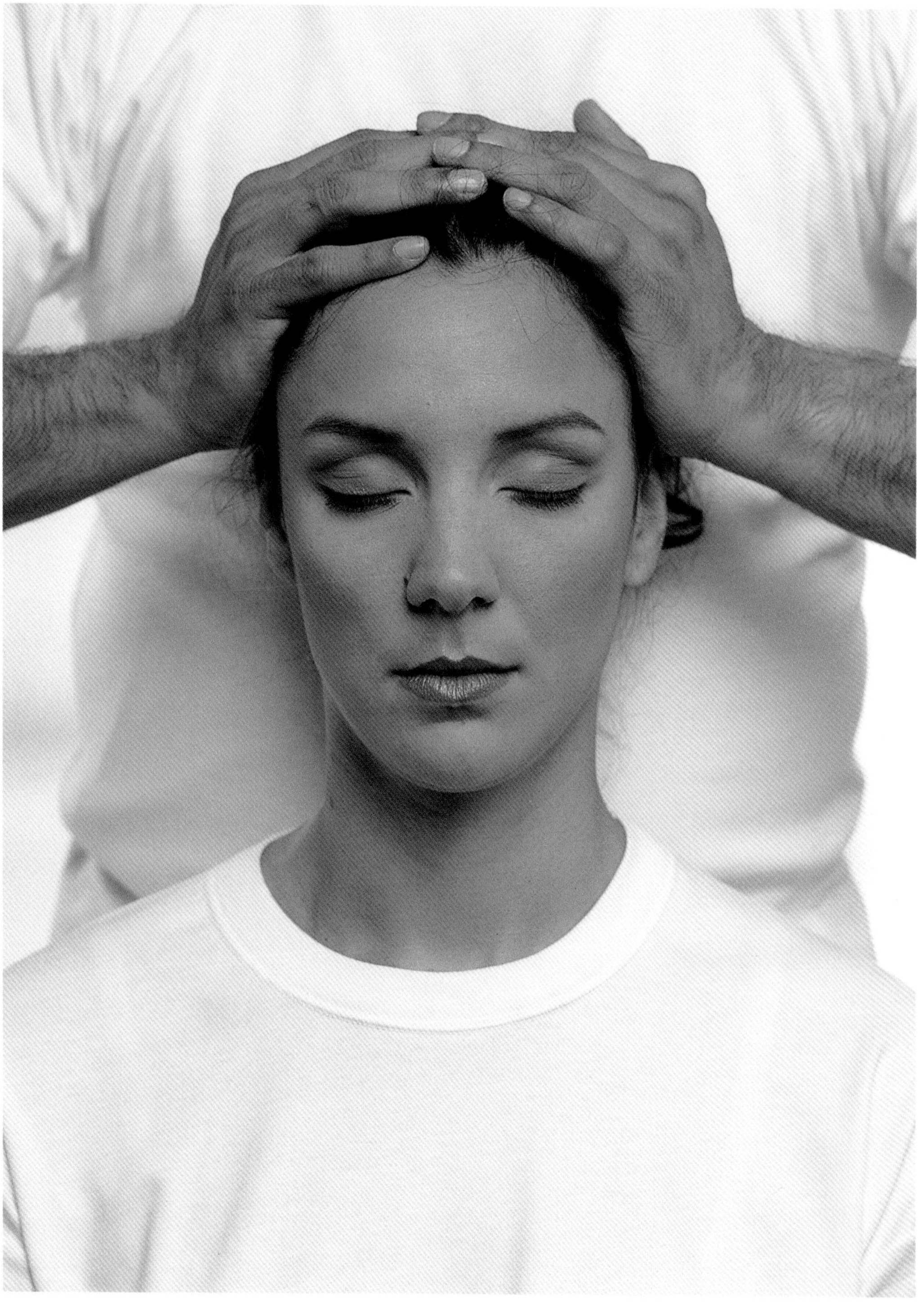

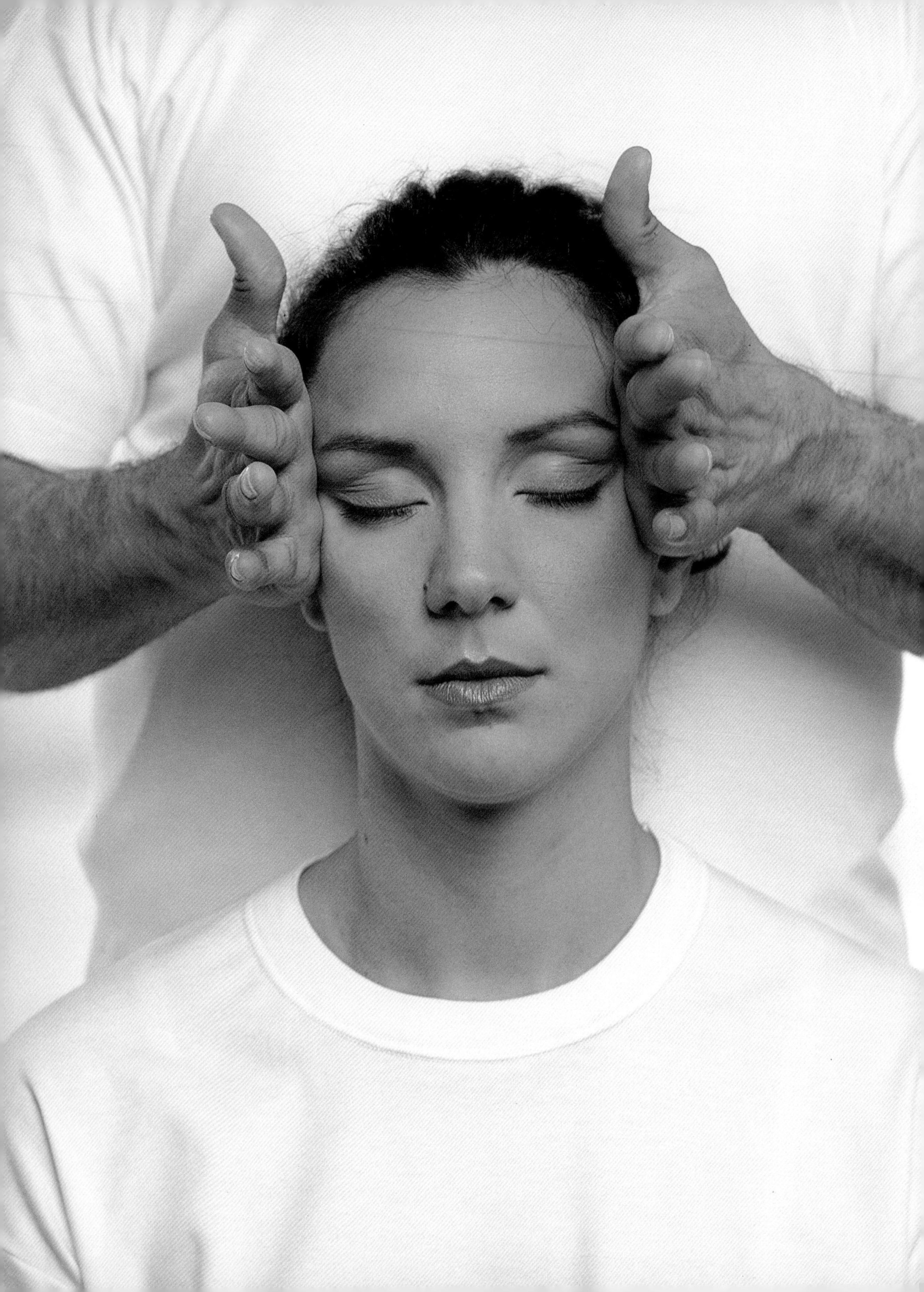

## CIRCULAR TEMPLE
## FRICTION

◆ Make sure you do not tilt the
head too far back as this could be very
uncomfortable for the other person.

◆ Stand close to the person you are
massaging and support their head with
your body. Place the heels of your hands
in front of the ears and the palms over the
temples. Use the palms of your hands to
make slow, wide, circular movements.
Remember this is a friction movement.

◆ This movement is excellent for
tension headaches in the temple area
and wonderful for relieving eyestrain.

'The ostrich burying its head in the
sand does at any rate ... convey
the impression that its head is the most
important part of it.' Katherine Mansfield

### RELAX THE FACE

◆ Lay your hands on the face with the palms of your hands over the cheeks, then gently trail your fingers up and down the face, giving the warmth of your healing hands. Repeat this movement several times.

### HEALTHY BODY

Combined with regular head massage the following will help you to combat stress.

• Exercise regularly to keep fit.

• Eat a healthy balanced diet with plenty of fresh fruit and vegetables.

• Stop smoking and limit alcohol consumption.

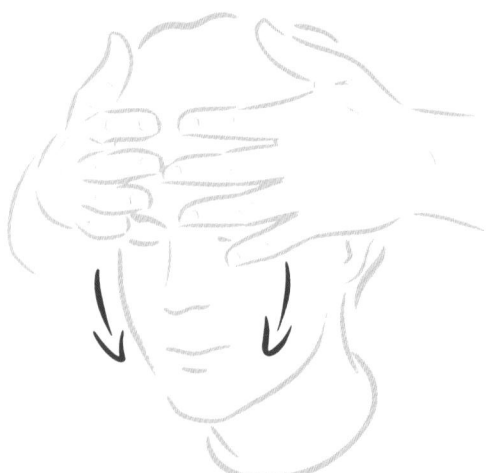

'Nothing makes as much difference as the expression on our faces.'

## FINAL SCALP MASSAGE

◆ Use your imagination! Combine some of the moves that you know the other person especially likes. Be gentle: they may be asleep! Finish off your Indian head massage with some wonderfully relaxing stroking movements. Finally, when you are ready to end the massage, lay your hands again on the other person's head in the same way as you did when you began the massage.

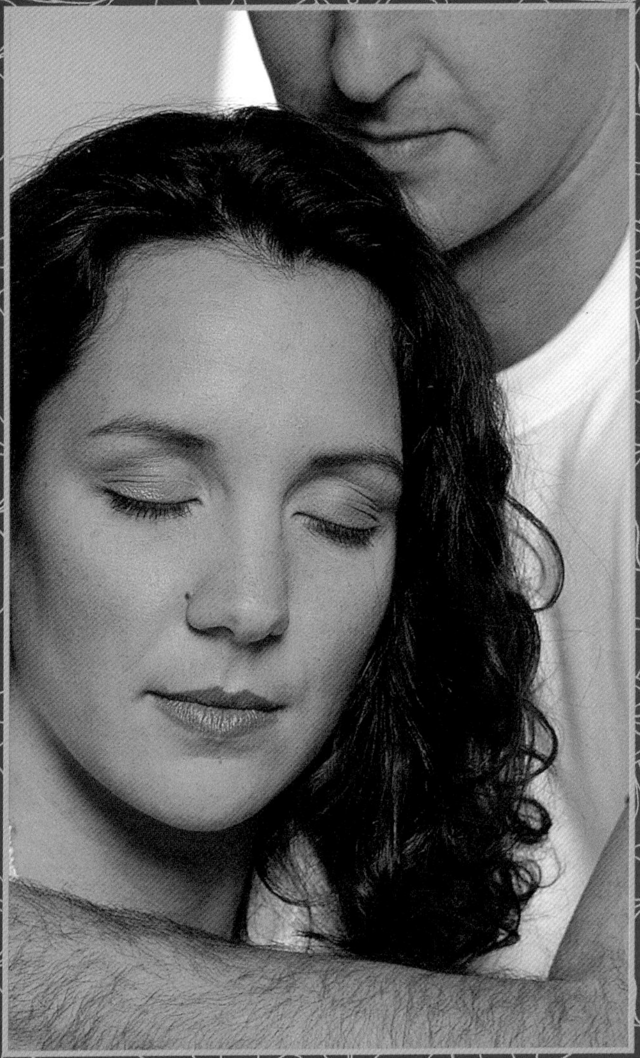

# CHAPTER 4

# Partners and Lovers

Head massage not only relieves tension, combats stress and improves the health of your hair: it can enhance your love life too! Head massage creates a special bond between you and your partner or lover that will bring you closer. If you haven't got a partner at the moment, spend time practising on friends or relatives. It will give you an added string to your lovemaking bow when the time comes.

# INTRODUCTION

Touching makes one feel nurtured, cared for and loved. A loving touch can relieve pain, soothe sorrow and promote health and general well-being. Most of us use touch instinctively – we may touch our lover's arm, kiss them or hold hands to show affection without thinking about it. However, as our culture has become more sophisticated, we have become more inhibited about our bodies and, as a result, touch each other less. Yet touch is one of the most vital ways of communicating; of giving and receiving. A caring massage creates feelings of trust and joy and connects you with your partner on a deep physical, spiritual and emotional level. If you and your partner take time to massage each other regularly, your bodies will become more sensual and receptive and you will feel more deeply in tune with each other. You may want to work on your partner's bare skin for this massage, and use sensual aromatherapy oils to heighten the erotic effect.

As the head, face and neck store a great deal of the anxiety, emotion and tension that accumulates in everyday life, touching these areas through massage will help to melt away troubles and open the paths of communication and understanding. If people massaged each other's head and hair on a regular basis, the world would be a happier and more loving place. The head and hair are extremely sensitive as the face and scalp are crowded with nerve endings. This makes them extremely receptive to touch. Massaging the head and hair is soothing, sensuous and deeply relaxing.

# SETTING THE SCENE

You may be in a hurry to begin, but it is important to set the scene before you start. This will help to relax you both. It is just as important for you to feel relaxed as it is for your partner, as any tension in your body may be felt by your partner or lover during the massage.

First of all, find a room where you know you will not be disturbed – don't be afraid to lock the door if necessary. The last thing you want is to be interrupted. Think about where your partner is going to sit, and make him or her as comfortable as possible. With a bit of imagination rugs, throws, drapes and cushions can transform an everyday room into an exotic sanctuary. Choose natural fabrics such as cotton and silk or luxurious velvet in sensual colours: reds, oranges and purples. These colours stimulate the lower chakras and waken your dormant sexual energy. Buy lengths of fabric or Indian saris, or make do with rugs, scarves and throws that you already have. Buy some flowers to delight your lover's eye: choose romantic roses with their heady scent or your partner's favourite. If you're feeling really extravagant, you could scatter the petals around the room.

After a busy day, soft lighting will impart a feeling of serenity and peace, so dim the lights: avoid an overhead light and use sidelights or, if possible, candles. Candles are a perfect complement to an oil burner to transform the mood of the room, and will help to create an atmosphere that will soothe and relax. You could also put on some soft, soothing music that both of you like – you don't have to perform the massage in silence. Music can contribute to a relaxing atmosphere and will provide a welcome contrast to the noise and bustle of the outside world. Make sure the room has no draughts and is pleasantly warm: too hot or too cold and neither of you will be able to concentrate on the massage. Finally, choose some essential oils to burn in an oil burner to create a subtle fragrance in the room: above all else, fragrance will assist in creating a sensual ambiance. If you are thinking of using essential oils to add to a base oil as part of the massage, choose ones to burn that are the same or complement them. I give suggestions on which essential oils to choose on page 73.

# BEFORE YOU BEGIN

Stroke-by-stroke instructions come later. First, you need to be aware of just how powerful Indian head massage can be when you follow my instructions. This massage should be featherlight and rhythmic. The gentle, repetitive moves will release your partner from the day's stress. You, your hands and your imagination will seduce your partner into the most magnificent of mellow, loving moods.

Remember to make sure your hands and nails are clean and that your hands are warm – cold hands on your partner's head will certainly not help to induce a state of relaxation. Run your hands under hot water to warm them up before you touch your partner. Ask your partner to remove any items of jewellery or spectacles that could get in the way of the head massage. Your partner will also need to remove all articles of clothing worn on the top half of the body if you are going to be using oils during this massage. Better still, remove them yourself! You will need to have a towel ready in case you spill any oil.

## Sensual Oils

The combination of head massage and fragrant oils will transport your partner into the realm of bliss. Try and use your partner's favourite aromatic oil. A sensual, relaxing aroma will definitely help to enhance the effect of your wonderful and loving massage. If you're going to use essential oil with your massage then think ahead and have the oils ready-mixed with the top of the bottle unscrewed so that you don't break the rhythm during the course of the massage to grapple with a bottle stopper. The oil should be warm – stand the bottle in a bowl of warm water for a few minutes first. Have a towel to hand in case of any spills. The oil should be made up of a base oil, which could be almond, sunflower or sesame, with a few drops of essential oil added. The best aphrodisiac oils are sandalwood, patchouli, musk, rose, jasmine, clary sage and ylang ylang. Combine two of these or add a spicy, stimulating oil such as cardamom, ginger, cinnamon or coriander. Alternatively, use any other aromatic oil of your partner's choice. Always blend the essentials oils with a base oil: essential oils are extremely concentrated and should never be used direct on the skin. Store the oils in pretty, dark glass bottles to enhance their look and preserve their properties.

## GETTING STARTED

Your partner should sit at a height where it is comfortable for you to reach both their shoulders and scalp. He or she should have their feet flat on the floor, hands in their lap and shoulders back. Above all they should feel calm and comfortable. You should stand squarely behind him or her, or sit on a chair and have your partner sit in front of you.

Before you apply the oil try a few warm-up moves. Tell your partner to close their eyes and let their imagination run wild while you massage them. You can begin by stroking your partner's hair and head, then slowly and softly massage your partner's ears. These are sensual areas and touching them gently helps your partner to get into a really loving mood. Next, softly stroke your partner's face up and down and side to side and then go back to the ears. Play with them. Return to the top of your partner's head. Stroke the hair gently with both hands, making maximum contact. Your hands should feel like waves, with no sense of beginning or ending. For a dramatic change of focus, continue stroking all over your partner's head, but this time use your fingernails to stroke the hair down the neck and continue down your partner's back. Who said head massage was exclusively about heads! This will make your partner feel fantastic.

**An important word of caution: this massage should not be performed if your partner has psoriasis, weeping eczema or any cuts or swelling on the scalp or face.**

# SHARING THE SENSUAL MASSAGE

Massage should always start and finish by laying your hands on your partner's head and holding them very lightly. Place the base of your palms above the ears, fingers facing forwards. This sets the mood at the beginning of the massage by sharing your energy with your partner. Then, after the massage, it makes your partner feel cared for and protected. We all have healing hands. Some people use the power in their hands and some people don't. As most tension accumulates in the shoulders and neck, your partner may experience some slight discomfort when these areas are treated. For this reason, begin with the shoulders, so that by the time you reach the final head stroking movements, your partner will be relaxed and any pain or discomfort will be forgotten.

Now here come the detailed instructions for this loving and sensual version of Indian head massage. You'll find more detailed information on the techniques in Chapter 3. Gently lay your hands on the top of the head and hold them there for around 30 seconds. Take three slow, deep breaths yourself (breathing in and out through your nose). This establishes a connection between you and your partner and puts him or her at ease.

If you are going to use the oil apply it now. Pour a few drops of oil on to your palm and gently rub it on the top of your partner's head. Take some more oil on your palm and then rub it between both hands and apply it to your partner's head and hair, working up towards the crown. Make sure the oil is evenly spread over the head.

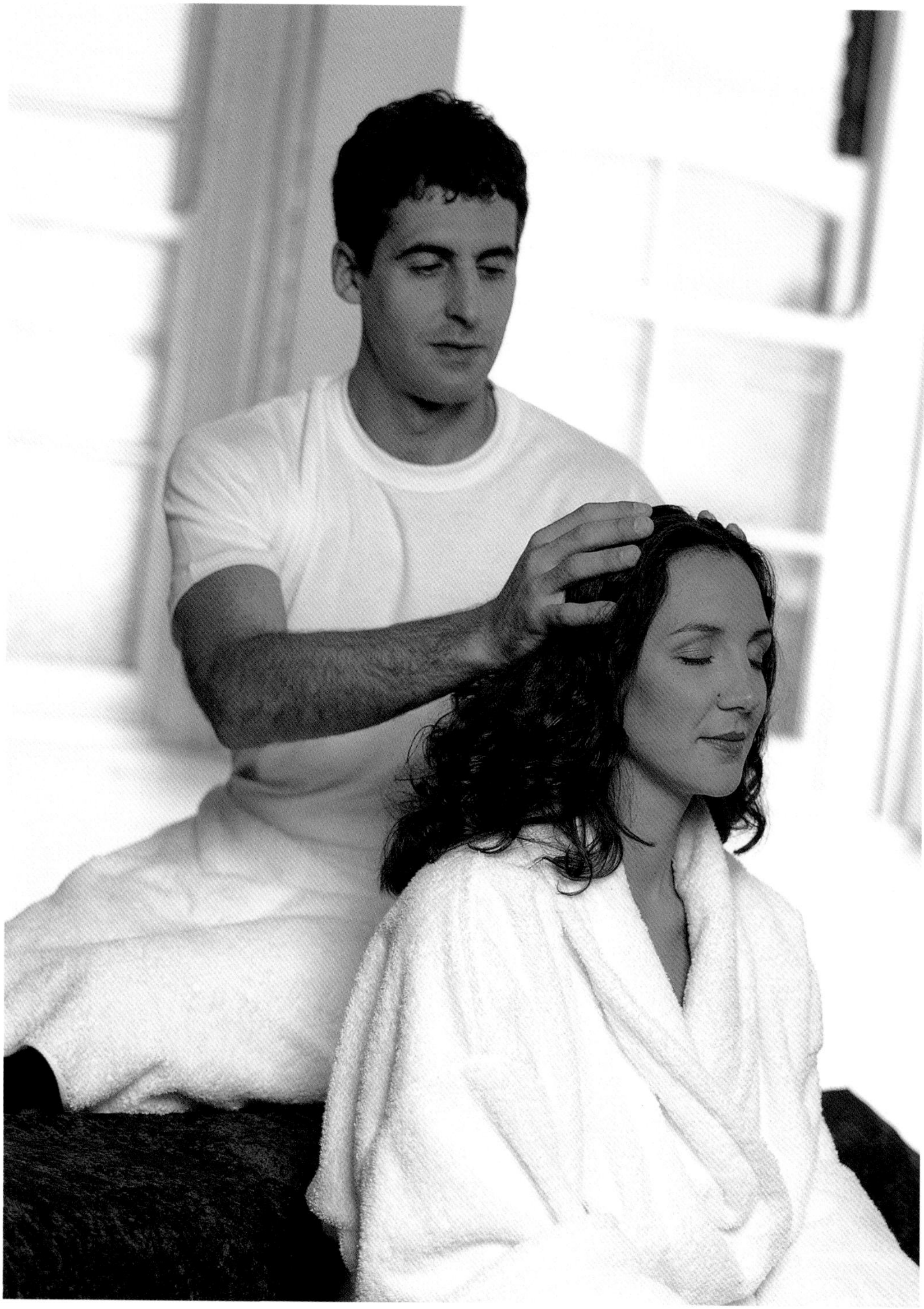

## STROKING

◆ Using both hands, one after another, gently stroke from the front to the back of the head, using long, sweeping movements with the whole of the hands. Use very light pressure. This should be followed by running your fingernails through the hair, then down the neck and the back. Work all round the head.

◆ This action relaxes the scalp and gives your partner a lovely tingly feeling.

## RUBBING THE BACK

◆ With the whole of your hand, rub briskly all over the back, using light pressure.

◆ This will warm your partner's back and relax him or her.

'Be in your fingers and hands as if your whole being, your whole soul, is there.' Osho

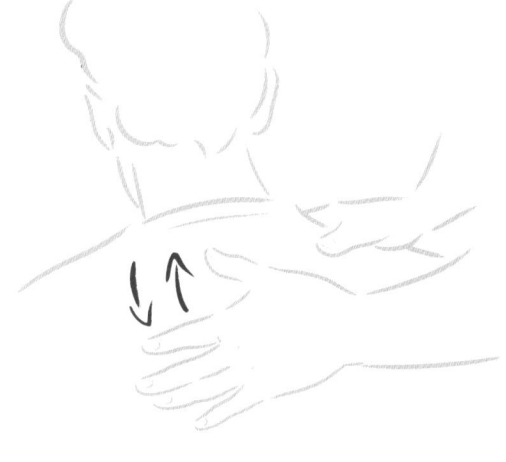

## AROMATIC OILS

• Sandalwood – Meditative, stress-relieving.

• Patchouli – exotic, uplifting and sensual.

• Lavender – purifying and relaxing, good for dry skin.

• Ylang ylang – excellent for impotence and frigidity: an aphrodisiac.

## HEEL ROLL ON THE SHOULDERS

◆ Place the thumb or heel of your hand just above the corner of the shoulder. Roll your thumb or heel forwards, using medium pressure, up and over the shoulder muscles. Repeat at the middle of the shoulder, then again at the junction of neck and shoulders.

◆ This will help to increase circulation and relieve stress and tension in your partner's shoulders. Use the heel of your hand, rather than the thumb, when your partner's shoulders are broad. This will allow you to exert more pressure, over a wider area, without getting tired.

## HEEL SQUEEZE ON THE SHOULDERS

◆ Reach from one side of your partner across to their other shoulder, placing one of your arms across their front and the other across their back. Squeeze their shoulder muscle with the heels of your hands using medium pressure. Do this in several places along the shoulder. Repeat a few times.

◆ This will soften tight muscles and release toxins.

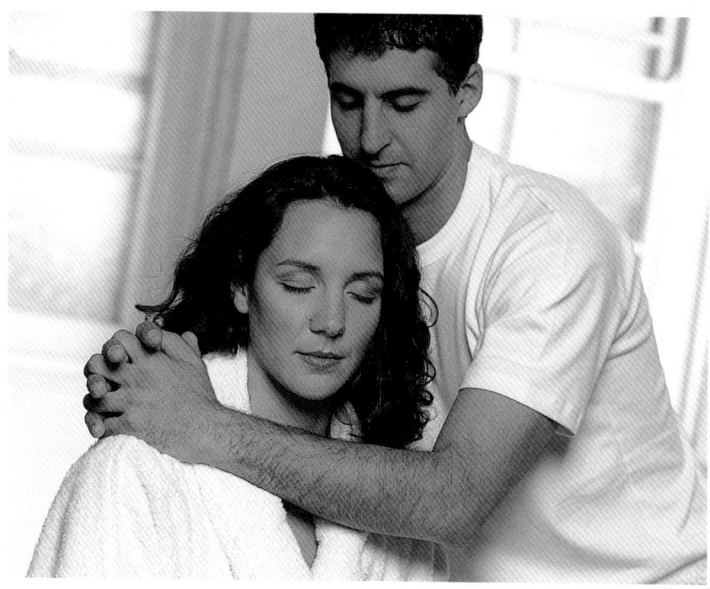

## CHAMPI ACROSS THE SHOULDERS

◆ Place your hands together in a prayer position, keeping your wrists relaxed. Make quick light hitting movements with your little fingers across the shoulders – touching the muscles only.

◆ This will stimulate the blood circulation.

## IRONING DOWN

◆ Iron down the upper arms (see page 46), using the heel of your hand to relax and loosen the arm muscles. Work from the top of the arm down to the elbow using the palms and heels of your hands with medium to deep pressure. Go down the sides of the arms then down the front and back of the arms. Repeat twice more.

## GIVING AND RECEIVING

Massage is a wonderful way to share time and emotion with your partner. It can soothe tension and misunderstanding and reinforce feelings of tenderness and intimacy. Together you can participate in a cycle of mutual giving and receiving.

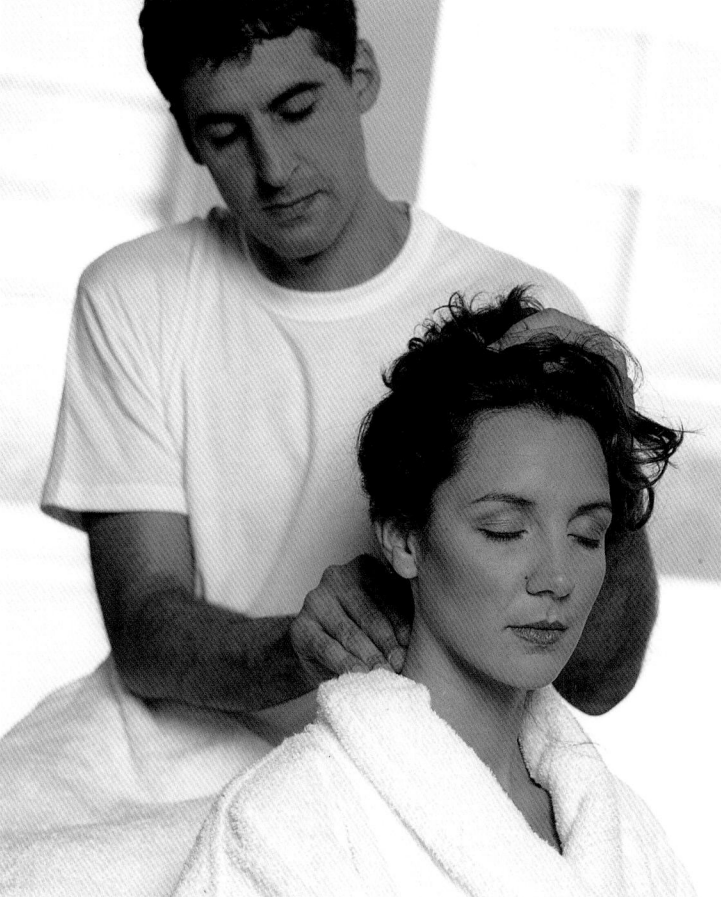

## HEEL ROLL

◆ Place your hands on top of the arm over the deltoid muscles. Place your fingers in front and the heels of your hands behind. Roll your heels over the muscles to arrive at your fingertips. Repeat at the middle of the upper arm. Repeat just above the elbow, then repeat twice more.

## NECK MASSAGE

◆ With one hand on the top of the head, tilt the head slightly back and with the other hand spread your thumb and fingers across the base of your partner's neck. Using firm contact with the skin, slide your hands up the neck, grasp the flesh and pull back. Grasp at the middle of the neck and pull back. Finally, grasp at the base of the neck and pull back. Repeat this a few more times.

◆ This is a soft tissue mobilization move, which loosens up the neck muscles.

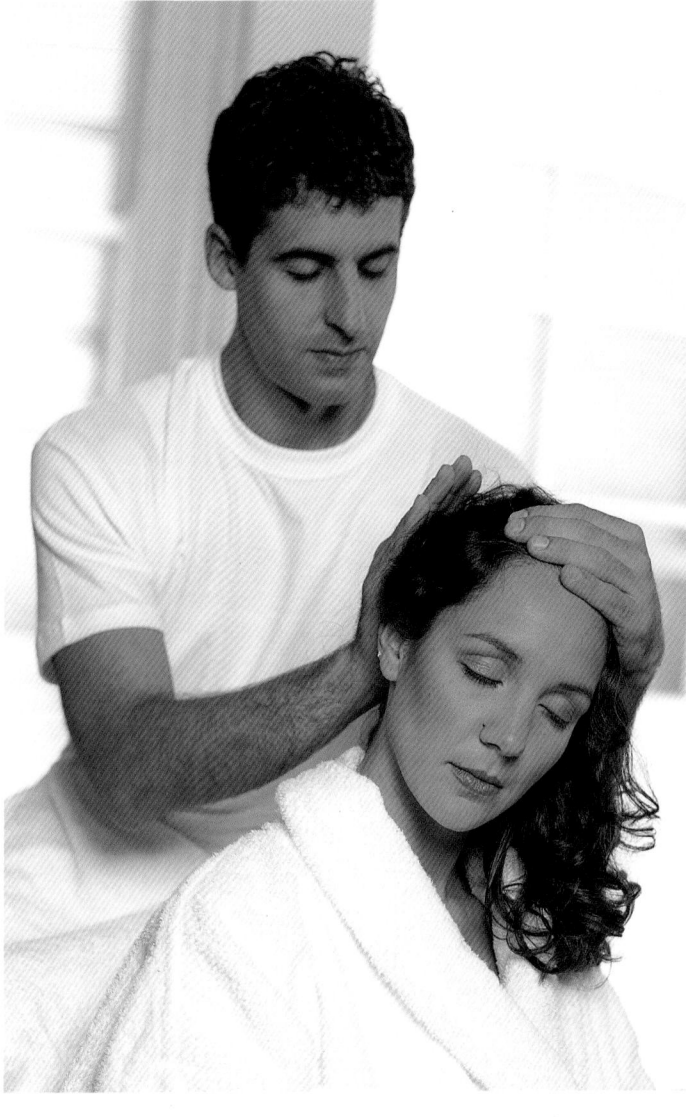

## HEEL RUB UNDER THE BACK OF THE HEAD

◆ With one hand supporting the forehead, place the heel of the other hand under the back of the head, pushing the fingers through the hair. Rub quickly and lightly up and down right across the back of the head.

◆ This helps to relieve tension in the muscles at the top of the neck and can often relieve tension headaches.

## BASE OILS

• Coconut – wonderful smell and excellent conditioning properties.

• Almond – popular and readily available.

• Sesame – excellent general purpose oil.

• See also page 109.

## SEDUCTIVE OILS

The popularity of aromatherapy and aphrodisiac essential oils may have enjoyed a recent boom, but their properties have been appreciated for centuries. Cleopatra is said to have used essential oils of jasmine and rose to seduce Mark Antony.

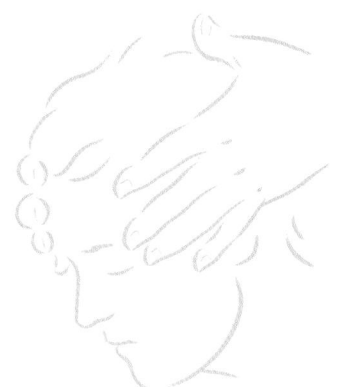

'By reciprocal indulgence,
their love endures.'

Kama Sutra

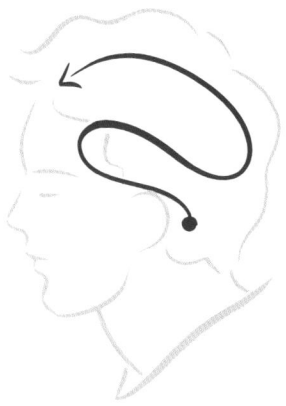

## SCALP RUB

◆ Support your partner's head with one hand and, using the palm of the other hand, carry out a swift, gentle rubbing movement as if you were washing a window. Start behind the ear, go around it and then away from the ear and up to the top of the head. Repeat the movement on the other side of the head.
◆ This relaxes and warms the scalp.

## HAIR RUFFLING

◆ Taking the hair between your fingers, ruffle the hair all over the head.
◆ This creates a very pleasing sensation.

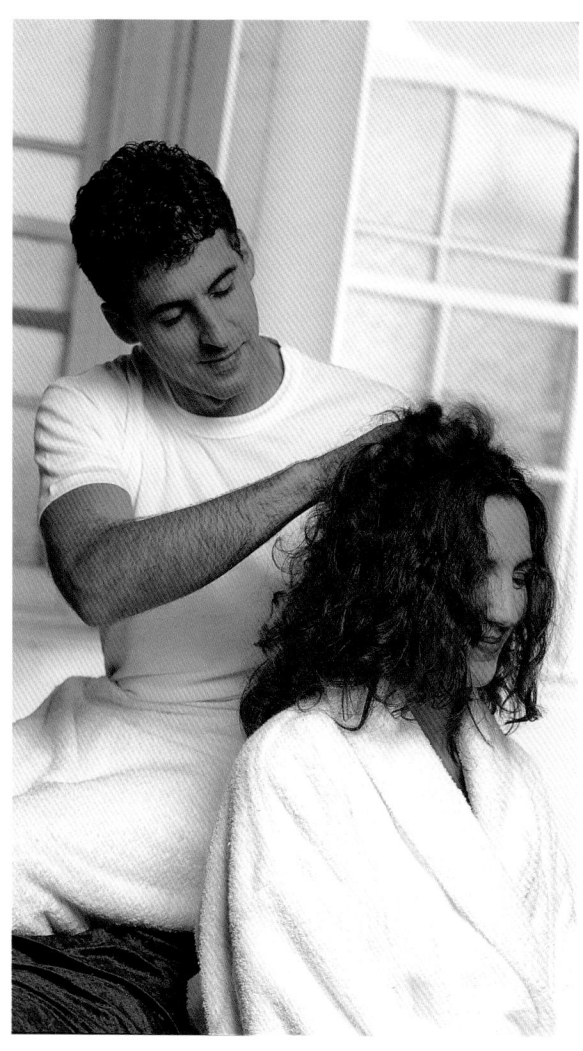

## HACKING ON THE HEAD

◆ Hold both hands over your partner's head, fingers facing forwards and palms facing inwards. Use the fingers of alternate hands to make quick, light hitting movements over the top of the head. Continue for a few minutes, making sure that you cover the whole area of the head.

◆ This pleasantly stimulating technique boosts the circulation and will leave your partner feeling relaxed and refreshed.

## 'If anything is sacred the human body is sacred'

### Walt Whitman

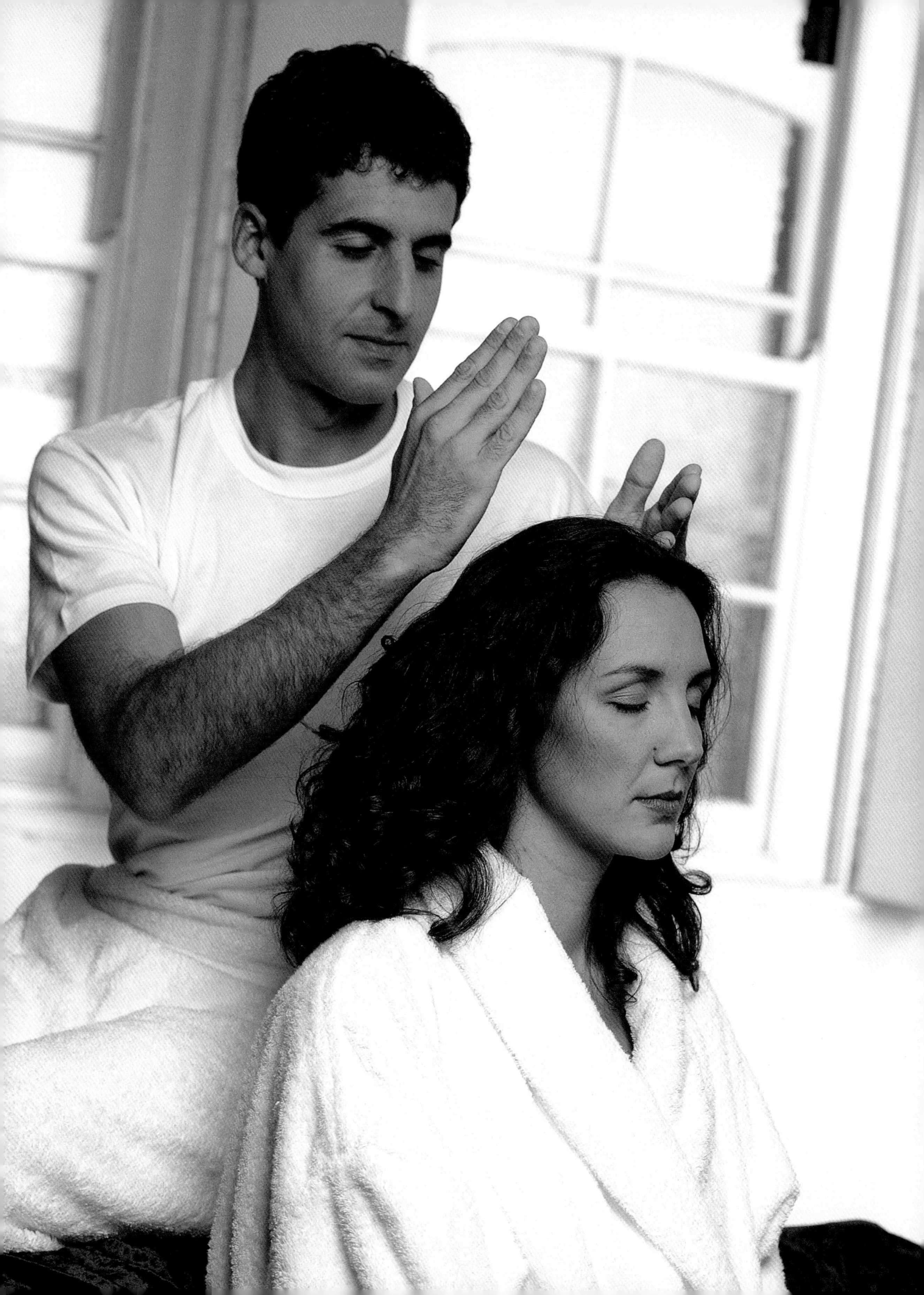

'It is a feeling which I can only describe as akin to a session of relaxation induced by hypnosis or one of those all too rare totally refreshing night's sleep where you wake up with the sensation that the world is a wonderful place.' The Entertainer

## GATHERING AND TUGGING THE HAIR

◆ Push your fingers through the hair on either side of your partner's head. Start either at the base of the head or the top of the head. Curl your fingers round into fists, keeping the back of your fingers against the scalp and getting hold of as much hair as you can. Gently tug on the hair. Continue all over the head. If your partner has short hair, then approach this from the top, grasping as much hair as possible. Continue in this way until you have covered the whole head.

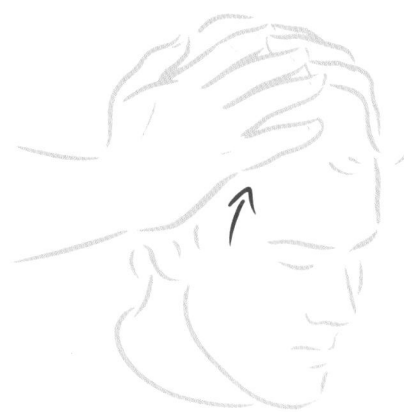

## HEAD SQUEEZE AND LIFT

◆ If your partner suffers from tension headaches, then this technique is ideal.

◆ Place the heels of both your hands just above your partner's ears, letting your fingers drop on to the top of the head like a cap. Squeeze with the heels, applying medium pressure, then lift the scalp and hold for a couple of seconds before letting go. Repeat the same move slightly in front of the ears. You can repeat it two or three more times.

◆ This will help to relieve most headaches and it has a calming effect.

## STROKING

◆ This is a repetition of the stroking movement above: using both hands, one after another, gently stroke from the front, using long sweeping movements with the whole of the hands. Use very light pressure. This should be followed by running your fingernails through the hair down the neck and right down the length of the back. Work all round the head.

◆ This action relaxes the scalp and stimulates the circulation, giving your partner a lovely tingly feeling.

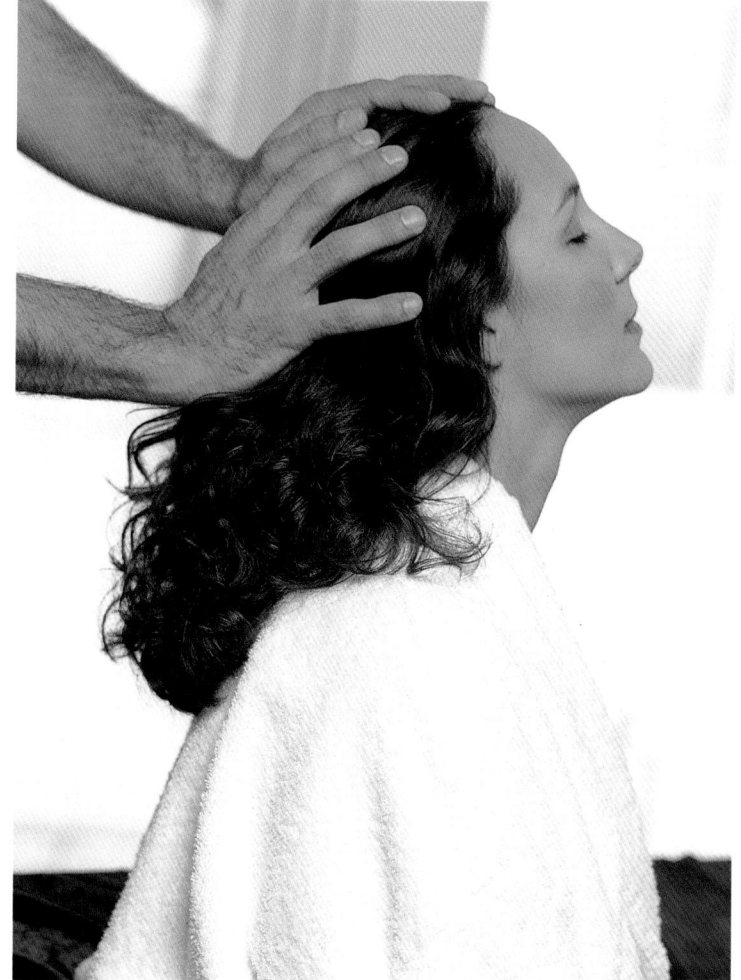

## EAR MASSAGE

◆ Position yourself either directly behind or in front of your partner. Place your flattened palms on your partner's ears and cover them entirely. Rub your flattened palms up and down and then in a circular movement using very light pressure. Your partner is guaranteed to find this particularly sensual.

◆ Gently squeezing between the thumb and forefingers, work your way up on the outer part of the ears and then down inside the ears two or three times.

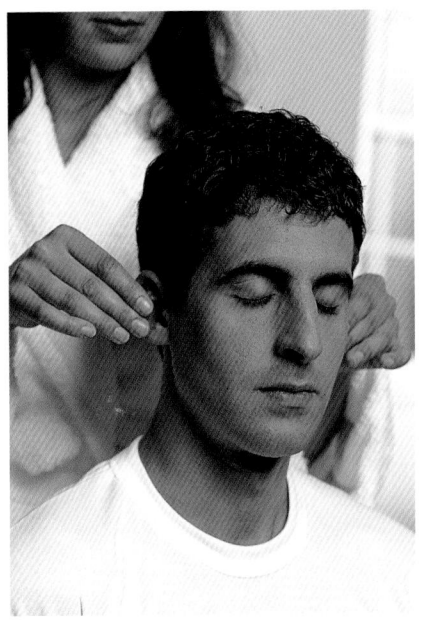

'... a regular dose of head massage can help cement a relationship.' Daily Mail

## POWER POINTS

Your ears contain a high concentration of nerve endings and are especially sensitive. Nibbling on your lover's ear is a well-know trick, but ear massage is particularly sensual and will give your partner a wonderful feeling.

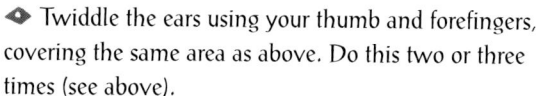

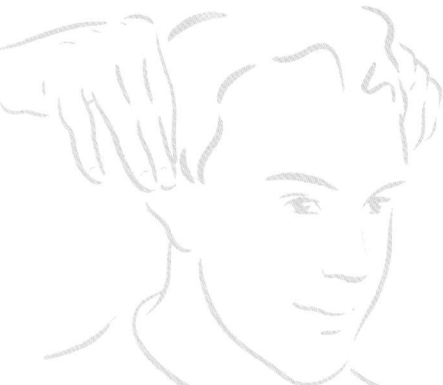

PULL THE EARS UP

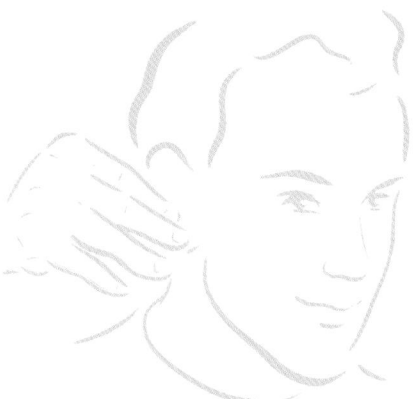

PULL THE EARS DOWN

◆ Twiddle the ears using your thumb and forefingers, covering the same area as above. Do this two or three times (see above).

◆ Pull the ears gently up and down.

◆ Flick the ears.

◆ By now your partner's ears will be red hot! He or she will feel tingly all over the ears and the face as the energy rushes down their whole body.

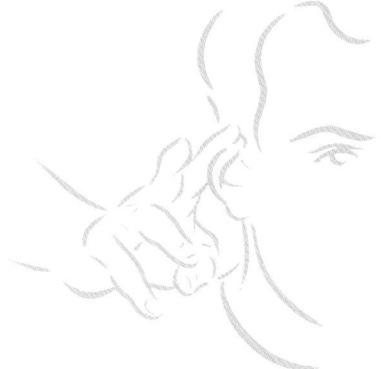

FLICK THE EARS

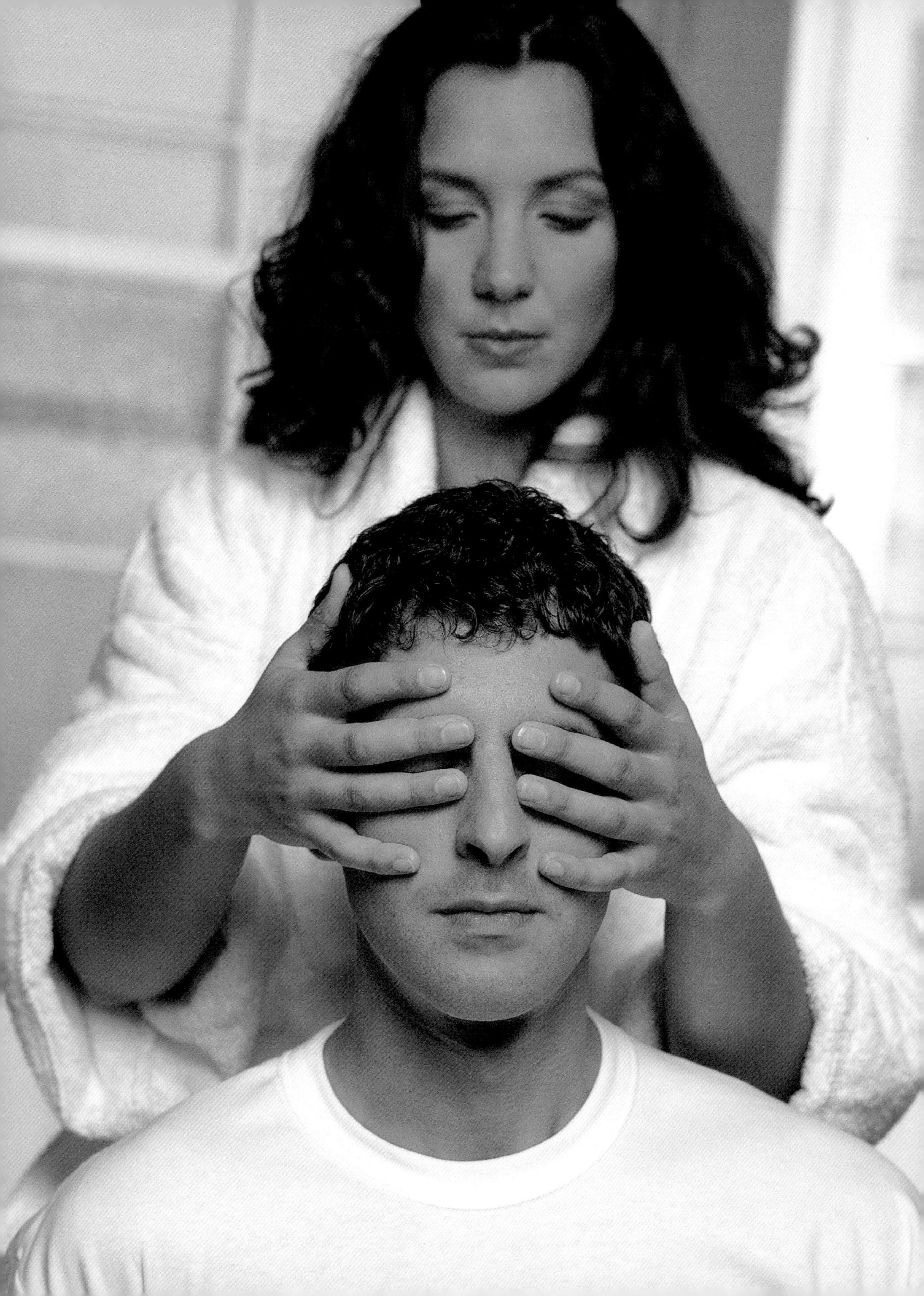

# GENTLE FACE MASSAGE

◆ First stroke lightly up and down, and then side to side on either side of the face, using the entire surface of your hands. With the palm against the face, move slowly down from the forehead to the chin. You can repeat this movement as many times as you like.

◆ Next, place your hands on your partner's cheeks. With your fingers facing the centre of your partner's face, hold the position for about ten seconds. Breathe calmly and deeply.

◆ Repeat the same, placing your hands on your partner's forehead.

◆ Repeat the same again, placing your hands on top of your partner's head.

◆ This massage is wonderful for leaving a tired and tense face looking beautifully relaxed and tranquil.

'It is the common wonder of all men, how among so many millions of faces, there should be none alike.' Sir Thomas Browne

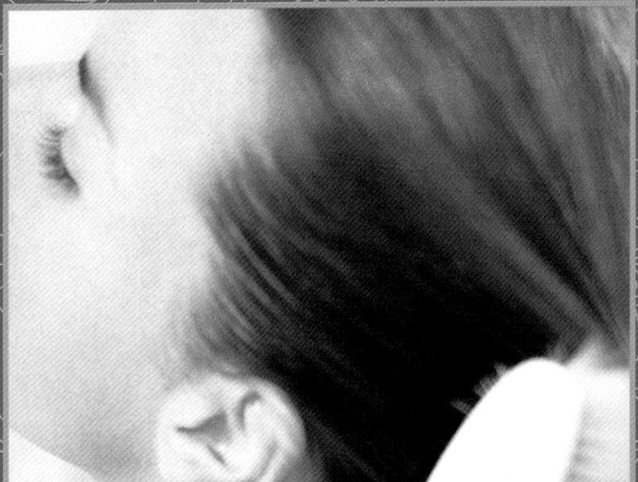

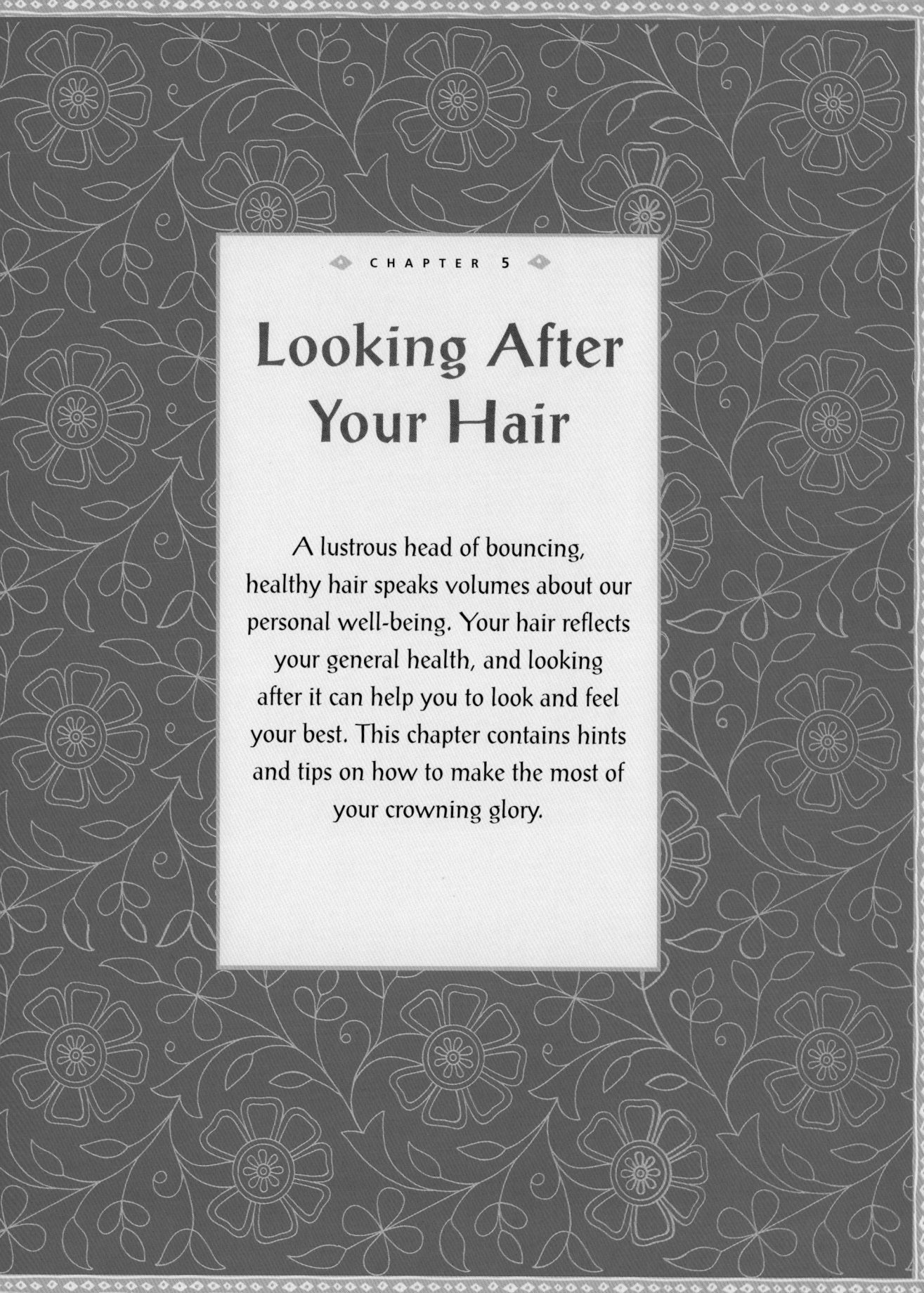

# CHAPTER 5

# Looking After Your Hair

A lustrous head of bouncing, healthy hair speaks volumes about our personal well-being. Your hair reflects your general health, and looking after it can help you to look and feel your best. This chapter contains hints and tips on how to make the most of your crowning glory.

# WHAT IS HAIR?

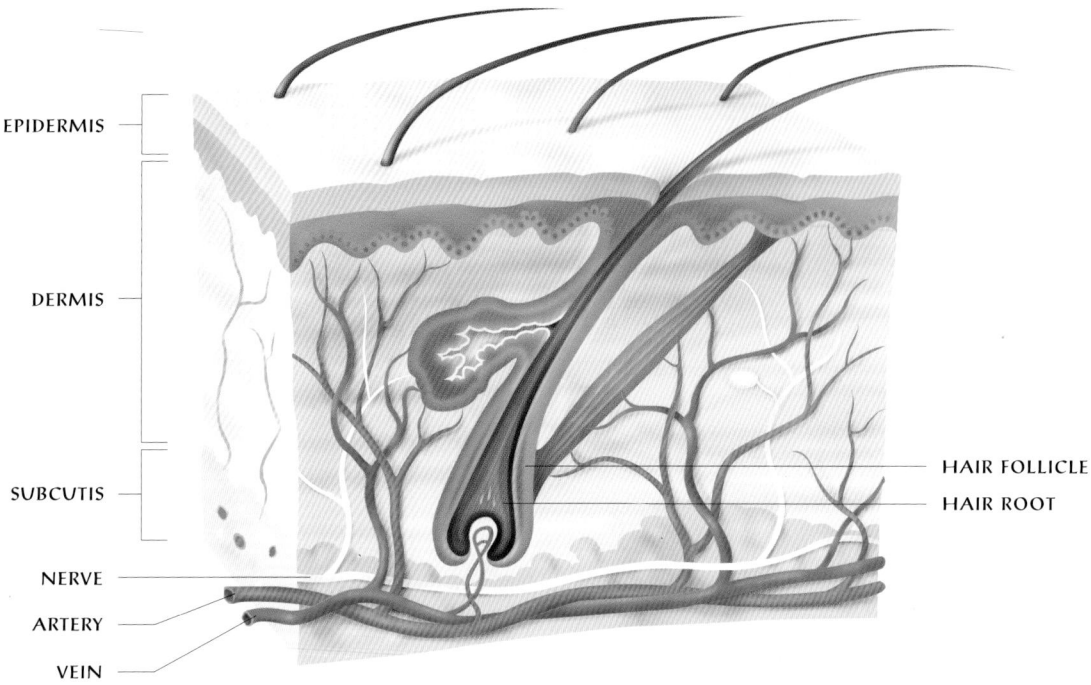

EPIDERMIS

DERMIS

SUBCUTIS

NERVE

ARTERY

VEIN

HAIR FOLLICLE

HAIR ROOT

Human hair is developed in relatively deep pits in the skin known as the hair follicles. These pits extend downwards below the entire thickness of the skin into the connective tissues. A baby's hair begins to appear about the third or fourth month of pregnancy and by about the sixth month the entire body is covered with a soft hair, known as lanugo, which is shed before birth. At birth, the hair of the scalp, eyebrows and eyelashes resembles the lanugo, but is thicker and stronger. During the first few months of babyhood these hairs are shed and replaced by permanent hair, which is hardier and thicker still.

The hair follicle is composed of two types of tissue; one originating from the skin and enveloping the hair root, and the other arising from the tissues below the skin where the blood enters and leaves the root from the general body circulation. In this way, nourishment is brought to the hair roots and waste products are removed. Any interference with this circulation will obviously upset natural growth.

Each hair root has a tiny muscle attached to it, which contracts under certain conditions and makes the hair stand erect. The muscle contracts when we are cold or frightened. With contraction and relaxation the hair is given exercise. Nervous conditions may cause prolonged contraction.

As the soft cells in the follicle multiply, each hair grows upwards from its bed. As the hair grows, it becomes stronger and harder and assumes its colour in accordance with the degree of general body pigmentation.

# TYPES OF HAIR

Hair comes in many different shades and textures:

- ◆ Coarse, tightly curled hair, characteristic of Negro races. This type grows in small tufts with tiny bald spaces between each tuft.

- ◆ Perfectly straight, thick hair which is nearly always black and belongs to Far Eastern races and the Indians of the Americas.

- ◆ Wavy, curly or smooth hair, characteristic of Europeans and Asians. It is mainly fair but can also be black, brown, red or tawny coloured.

- ◆ Frizzy, coarse-textured, usually dark hair common among Australian aborigines and people of mixed race.

Hair colour tends to be lighter in cold, northern countries and darker in hot, southern countries where extra pigment is needed in the hair and the skin to protect them from the effects of the sun.

# COMMON HAIR DISORDERS

## Greasy Hair and Scalp

This is caused by overactivity of the sebaceous glands (if these glands are underactive, the hair will become dry and brittle, and the scalp may develop dandruff). Frequent shampooing does not increase the amount of sebum, but it can dry out the scalp.

## Damaged Hair

Nearly all cosmetic procedures that are applied to hair can be damaging. Bleaching, drying, perming, straightening, even heated rollers, curling tongs and blow-drying can all cause the hair to become dry, break and split. In addition, many of the chemicals used can be irritant and cause contact dermatitis.

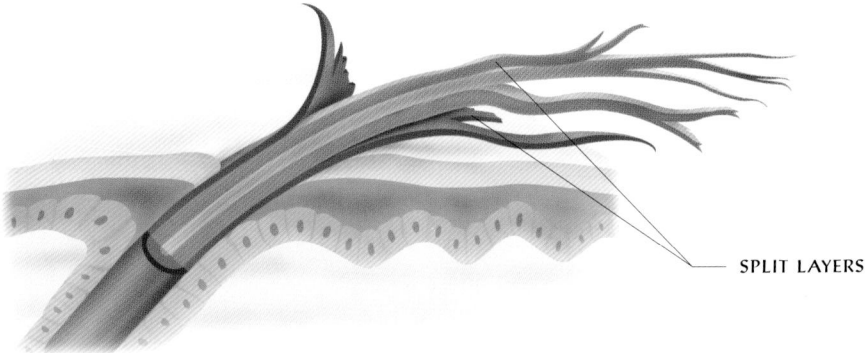

SPLIT LAYERS

## Dandruff

The scalp is a living organ. It gets rid of waste, but it also absorbs chemicals from any hair products used. One of the ways the scalp keeps itself healthy is to shed outer skin cells. When the shedding of the skin of the scalp becomes excessive and obvious, this is termed dandruff. It is normally the result of too little or too much sebum being secreted by the sebaceous glands in the skin. Dry white flakes are produced when there is too little sebum, and yellowish, oily, sticky flakes are a result of too much sebum.

Dandruff can also be the result of fungal infection, or may be produced by sensitivity to hair products. The body is so resilient that it can put up with irritants for years before it reacts. If you use hair dyes and styling products you should also use a gentle herbal shampoo to reduce chemical build-up on the scalp.

Hairspray which coats the hair in plastic and crumbles to powder when it is brushed also contributes to a flaky scalp. Medicated shampoos, based on antifungal agents, would seem to have little to offer. Some medicated shampoos contain harsh medications that are not particularly suitable for frequent use.

## Head Lice

Head lice are highly contagious. If your child becomes infected it is important to treat the problem as soon as possible, and to treat the whole family, including yourself, to prevent the lice from being passed backwards and forwards. There are many aromatherapy oils that kill head lice, for example, tea tree, eucalyptus, geranium, rosemary, thyme and lavender. Try 20 drops of tea tree oil, 10 of lavender and 15 of eucalyptus mixed together thoroughly in a base oil of almond or sesame. Massage into the scalp and leave on for a couple of hours, or overnight, before rinsing off with shampoo. If necessary, repeat this process every couple of days. You can also use lavender oil for scalp massage as a preventive measure.

## Hair Loss

Hair loss can occur for a number of different reasons. Most common of these is androgenetic alopecia, or male pattern baldness. This is a genetic disorder that can be passed on through successive generations by either parent.

Hair normally grows at the rate of 12mm a month, and each hair grows for up to five years before the follicle is exhausted and the hair falls out. The follicle then goes into a three month resting period before a successor is germinated. This process continues throughout a lifetime. However, androgenetic alopecia causes the hair to shrink in size, so that the hair becomes thinner and shorter, while the scalp between each hair becomes more and more obvious. This process can start any time after puberty and, according to the evidence, can only be slowed down, never reversed.

Although it affects both men and women, women are far less likely to develop full-blown alopecia because the gene reacts to the androgen range of hormones, which includes testosterone and is more prevalent in males. Oestrogen, the equivalent dominant hormone in women, keeps the action of the gene in check, at least until the menopause. However, a woman who carries the inherited alopecia gene may suffer progressive hair thinning as she gets older. Occasionally the hair may become very sparse and fine, especially on the front of the scalp. Again, this is due to changes in the levels of sex hormones, and often occurs after the menopause.

The age at which hair loss strikes is particularly significant for men. Hair loss from the temples may start soon after puberty, but the older a man is before he begins to lose his hair, the better the long-term prognosis is. If he can keep most of his hair until his late thirties, then he's likely to keep it well into old age. Although baldness often runs in families, it is not inevitable that balding parents will produce children who also lose their hair: there is only a 50% chance of the gene being passed on.

Scientists are looking for the gene responsible for causing inherited baldness. It may take some time for them to discover anything useful. However, baldness is often caused by other factors such as stress, severe shock, serious illness, surgery or radiotherapy. This manifests in three recognized conditions:

◆ Alopecia areata – hair lost in patches
◆ Alopecia totalis – all the hair lost from the head
◆ Alopecia universalis – total loss of all body hair

Alopecia areata begins with the sudden appearance of circular areas of baldness on the scalp or in the beard in men. These can sometimes join up to form one large patch. Time is the best healer. Hair growth normally returns within six to 12 months.

Stress has been known to cause severe hair loss, albeit usually temporary. When the source of the stress is removed the hair normally grows back quite naturally.

Most women lose some hair two or three months after having a baby. This is because hormonal changes during pregnancy prevent normal hair loss, so old hairs stay in the follicles and are lost all at once when hormones begin to revert to their previous levels.

Anaemia can also be a factor in hair loss, and extra iron taken on a regular basis may help, especially for women who suffer from heavy periods.

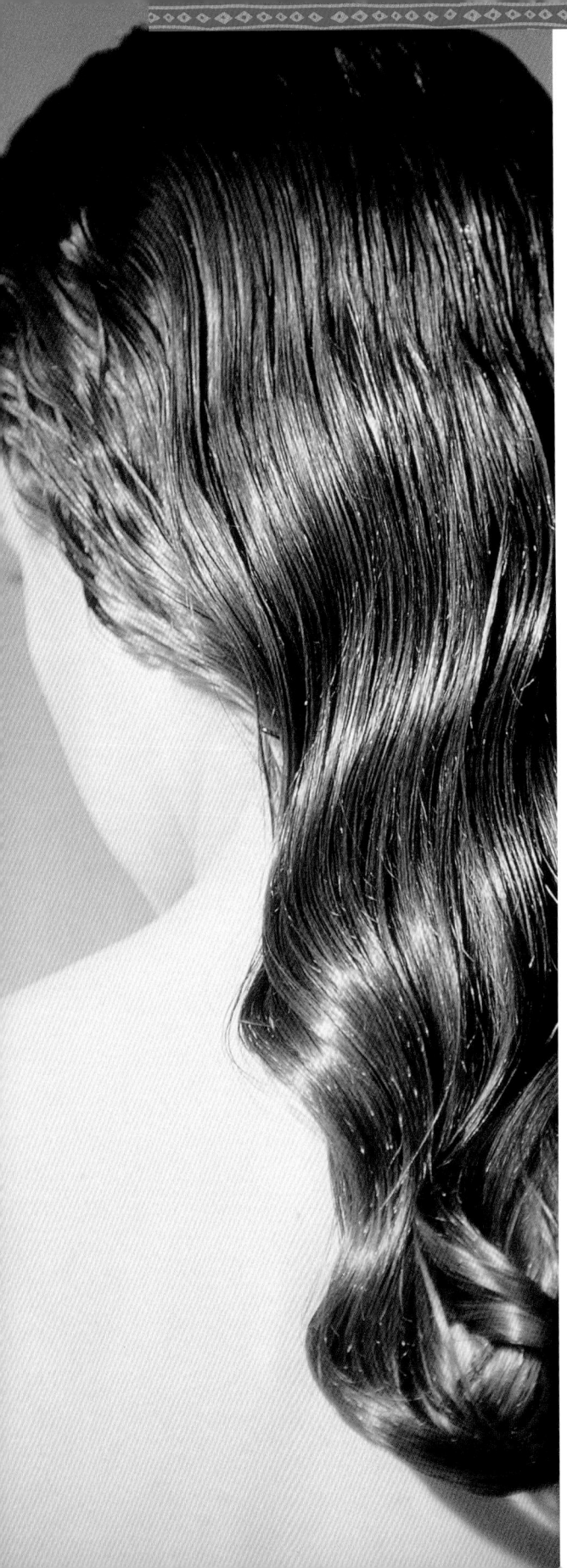

# Maintaining Healthy Hair

Hair, like skin, is a visible reminder of our state of health. When your body is working well on the inside, it looks good on the outside, but when stress, ill health or a poor diet get to work on the body, hair is often one of the first things to be affected. Dull, lank and brittle hair can all be symptoms of some neglected aspect of your general health as well as a consequence of how you treat your hair.

The structure of your hair records what is happening in your body. Some natural therapists analyse the minerals in hair to gain an idea of the mineral content of the body. Stress and hormonal changes also register in the hair, though the information is always slightly retrospective. If you go through a stressful period, you may not notice that your hair quality has changed until three months later.

The greatest favour you can do for your hair is to look after your health. A nourishing diet, frequent exercise and regular restorative sleep is what it takes to feed it from the roots. Loose muscles on the scalp will assist in better blood circulation. Regular Indian head massage strengthens the hair roots and improves the blood circulation under the scalp. As a result, the hair follicles become stronger. The special oils that can be used in massage (see 'Using Oils' page 108) are absorbed and provide

**The greatest favour you can do for your hair is to look after your health...**

nutrients to the roots. However, even if you do take care of your health and have regular head massage, you should also think carefully about how you treat your hair itself.

## Shampoos

One of the biggest enemies of hair is pollution. We're constantly perspiring and producing sebum. This attracts dirt and pollution that clings to the hair, so we need to wash our hair frequently to keep it in good condition. However, the harsh detergents in shampoo can strip our hair of its natural protective barrier. Try rinsing your hair with water instead of shampooing whenever possible, as this will wash out dirt without removing the natural protective oils. Shampoo and/or conditioner should not be used more than two or three times a week.

Strictly speaking, there are no natural shampoos, because all shampoos contain detergent. Companies that produce the most natural products use gentle detergents derived from natural materials, but even these are far too processed to be classified as natural. Shampoo also contains some preservatives to prolong the life of the product.

Look for a product that balances the effects of the detergent and preservatives with plenty of natural ingredients. Good quality shampoos that include lots of fresh herbal material have a conditioning effect and can improve hair quality. Essential oils can be beneficial in shampoos and conditioners, even if they are only left on the hair for a matter of minutes. Hair swells by up to 30% when it's wet, making it easier for products to penetrate the hair shaft. But if essential oils can be absorbed into the hair, so, in theory, can chemicals. Minimize the risk by choosing a shampoo that's high in natural ingredients and rinse your hair thoroughly after shampooing.

## WASHING YOUR HAIR

Always choose a gentle shampoo and shampoo only once using just a little of the product. Rinse well and use a suitable conditioner to reduce the risk of damage. Wrap your hair in a towel without wringing. Wet hair is easily broken, so comb the end section first, working up the hair shaft to the roots, using a wide-toothed comb. Heat damages hair because it dehydrates it. If you do use a hairdryer, wait until your hair has almost dried naturally before blow-drying – set on medium heat and hold the hair drier about 20cm (8 inches) away from your hair. The best way to get your hair dry is to allow it to dry naturally or to use a towel. It is not a good idea to dry it in the direct rays of the sun as this is liable to make the scalp scaly.

# Helpful Treatments

## Herbal Treatments

Herbal treatments have been used for centuries to treat disorders and improve the condition of hair. Try the following:

- An infusion of rosemary rubbed into the scalp is a general hair tonic.

- An infusion of comfrey should be used on dry hair, and lavender on oily hair: rub this in daily, but do not rinse it off.

- For dark brown hair try massaging sage tea well into the scalp daily. This is good as a final rinse after shampooing and will mask up to 5% of grey hairs.

- Blonde hair benefits from being rinsed in chamomile tea.

- Before shampooing rub a little almond oil into the scalp to prevent drying.

- You could also rub aloe vera gel into the scalp; leave this on overnight and then shampoo. This is a general tonic, but it may also reduce excess sebum.

- For hair loss, drink an infusion of clivers herb – 25g (1oz) to 0.5l (1pt) water in 45–60ml (3–4 tbsp) doses three times daily. Store this infusion in the fridge. Also, try the aloe vera gel (see above).

- For dandruff an infusion of sage, nettles or clivers should be massaged thoroughly into the scalp each day and be used warm as a final rinse when shampooing. The aloe vera gel (see above) may also be used.

## Homeopathy

Hair problems generally reflect the condition of the rest of the body. One therapy that treats the whole body, and not just specific symptoms is homeopathy. A homeopath may offer the following:

- Kali carbonicum for dry hair.

- Bryonia for greasy hair.

- Phosphoric acid for hair loss following periods of stress or the death of a friend or relative.

- Sepia when hair loss is associated with pre-menstrual depression or tension, and there is chilliness, weeping and irritability.

## Massage

Massage the scalp daily to increase the blood supply to the hair follicles, thus improving nutrition and removing impurities. Once or twice a week, massage with olive oil, coconut oil, sesame oil or home-made mayonnaise to condition the hair. Essential oils can be added to these base oils to treat specific hair conditions.

| Use | Oils |
| --- | --- |
| For greasy hair | clary sage, chamomile, lemongrass |
| For dry/damaged hair | ylang ylang, sandalwood, rosewood |
| For normal hair | geranium, lavender, rosemary |
| For light hair | lavender, lemon |
| For dark hair | sandalwood, patchouli, ylang ylang |
| As a rinse/tonic | rosemary, petitgrain, ylang ylang |
| For growth | juniper, rosemary |
| For an itchy scalp | cedarwood, tea tree |
| For dandruff | patchouli, tea tree |

## Naturopathy

Hair and scalp problems may reflect underlying imbalances of function or nutritional deficiencies; if you suspect that this is the case, you should seek professional advice from a qualified naturopath. He or she will advise you on how to adopt a wholefood diet excluding refined carbohydrates, dairy products and animal fats, and take an adequate amount of exercise.

- ◆ A naturopathic remedy for dandruff is to apply plain 'live' yogurt as a conditioner.

- ◆ Leave it on for at least 10 minutes and then rinse out ,afterwards wash the hair in the normal way.

- ◆ As a final rinse, use a strong infusion of nettle, thyme or sage plus 30ml/2 tbsp vinegar or lemon juice.

## Vitamin and Mineral Treatment

Certain vitamins and minerals are very beneficial for the health of your hair. Silica forms part of the starches that make up the hair's basic structure, so if your hair is damaged or fragile, it could be strengthened by taking a silica supplement. Silica is also important if you have brittle nails, prematurely ageing skin or eat a diet high in processed foods. Zinc supplements can help to improve hair quality and may be advisable if you take the Pill or are on hormone replacement therapy (HRT). Oestrogen lowers zinc levels and increases your need for the B vitamins, which are essential for healthy hair. B vitamins help to maintain hair colour and quantity, and prevent dandruff. Dandruff can also be caused by lack of essential fatty acids. Evening primrose oil and starflower oil supplements can help, especially if you have menstrual problems, or eczema in the hair line.

## Oils

For lifeless, dry, dull hair, try a head massage with a specially prepared Ayurvedic hair oil. This oil has a vegetable oil base, to which five different herbs, traditionally used in India for the treatment of hair are added. These herbs are sandalwood, henna and three others, not commonly used in this country, called brahmi, shikakai and amala. All five make the hair shiny, smooth and lustrous, encouraging hair growth and helping to combat dandruff and dry scalp disorders. The oil is available from the London Centre of Indian Champissage.

◆ Apply 5–15ml of the oil to damp hair and massage into the scalp and hair following the self-massage technique on page 111. Leave the oil in your hair for a minimum of 2 hours, and overnight if possible.

◆ Wash out with a herbal shampoo and finish with a herbal conditioner.

◆ For dry or chemically treated hair try the following mixture:

> 25ml virgin olive oil
> 10ml jojoba oil
> 10ml wheatgerm oil
> 3 ml essential oil blend: 8 drops geranium, 12 drops lavender, 6 drops patchouli

◆ Pour the vegetable oils into a clean 50ml bottle, add the essential oils and shake. Apply 5–15ml of the blend to damp, but not dripping, wet hair. Rub in and leave for 20 minutes.

◆ This treatment makes your hair very oily, but it does have a wonderful effect. When you come to wash your hair, it is easier to remove the oil if you rub a little shampoo into your hair and scalp before you wet it.

◆ Repeat the treatment twice a week for four to six weeks.

◆ For dandruff try:

     100ml jojoba or apricot oil (or mix the two)
     20 drops orange oil
     17 drops cedarwood oil
     17 drops patchouli oil
     10 drops tea tree oil

◆ Pour the oils into a bottle and shake the bottle vigorously. Massage the oil into the scalp and through the hair. Take care to keep the oil off your face as the mix is quite strong.

◆ Cover your hair with a towel and relax for a few hours. Shampoo and dry as normal.

◆ Do this twice a week if your dandruff is severe.

◆ Omit the tea tree oil and use once a week for mild cases of dandruff.

◆ Another effective treatment for dandruff is to cut a lemon in half, remove most of the juice and rub the two halves of peel all over your scalp.

'Regular head massage with natural vegetable oils keeps the hair strong and lustrous. Massaging the scalp stimulates the flow of blood to the follicles, bearing nutrients needed for healthy hair growth.' Harpers and Queen

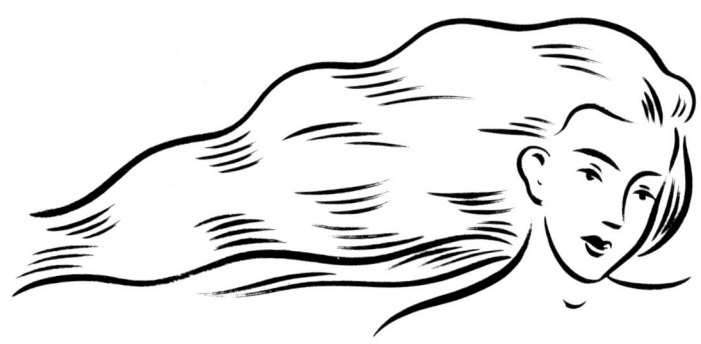

# Case Histories

Age:19
Sex: Male
Profession: Motorcycle courier

◆ Symptoms: Jim had severe dandruff. Six months prior to his first visit, he had had bronchial pneumonia. He was suffering from a heat rash. His girlfriend brought him to me, as she was worried about his increasingly violent bouts of temper. Jim had had a troubled childhood. He was clearly on edge and complained about headaches and pain in his sinuses.

◆ After the first treatment: During the treatment, Jim's shoulders felt ticklish but he stayed with it. I suggested to him that I use my special Ayurvedic oil, which would help his dandruff. As I calmed him down, he felt he wanted to talk.

◆ After subsequent treatments: Jim felt more grounded, relaxed and energized. His dandruff cleared up completely after four treatments with the oil.

◆ Recommendations: I recommended that he continue receiving Indian head massage once a week for a month and then review the situation.

Age: 31
Sex: Female
Profession: Journalist

◆ Symptoms: Janice came to me with hair problems. She had been losing quite a lot of hair for the past three months. She had tried various things but nothing had helped. Janice is a workaholic and constantly under stress at work. She had lots of deadlines to meet and was suffering from headaches.

◆ After the first treatment: After one treatment, Janice felt as though she had had a good sleep. In fact, she did nod off during the treatment! She felt very relaxed. I had used my Ayurvedic oil, as her hair was very dry and lanky. I asked her to come for five further treatments.

◆ After subsequent treatments: At the end of six treatments Janice said that when she washed her hair she was losing far less. She told me, with a degree of pride in her voice, that her colleagues at work had remarked that her hair looked healthier and shinier and asked her what she was using. She also said that she was feeling much more relaxed and could concentrate much better. She hadn't had a single headache since the start of the treatment.

◆ Further recommendations: I recommended that she should regularly massage her head with the special Ayurvedic hair oil and have professional head massage treatments whenever she can.

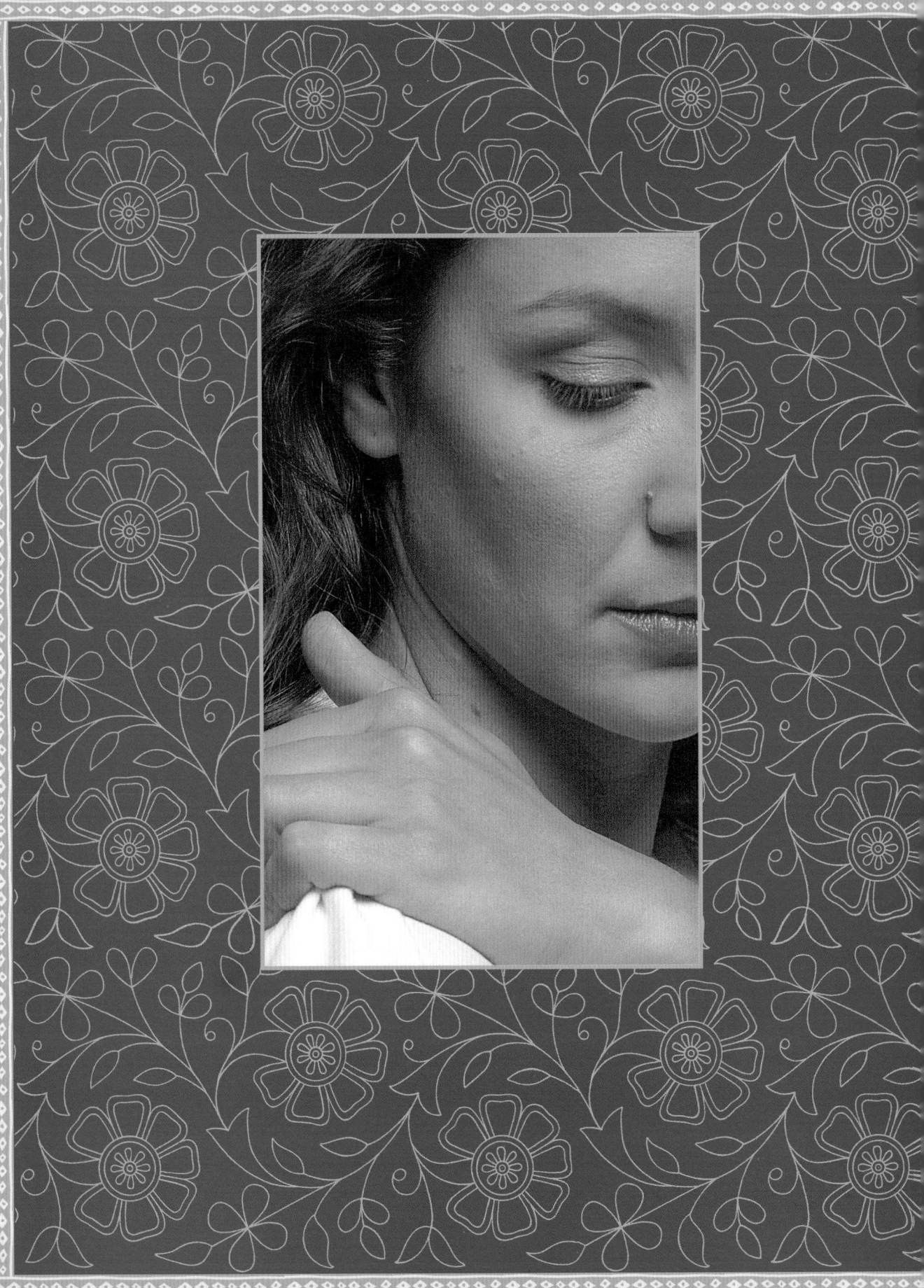

# CHAPTER 6

# Self Massage

Do you often come home from work feeling tired and worn out? Do you have periods when your energy levels are low and you lack enthusiasm for life? Do you long for someone to give you a nice, relaxing neck and shoulder massage? You don't need anyone with you to experience the benefits of a head massage: you yourself have the power to melt away pain and relieve stress in your own fingertips.

# Introduction

If there is nobody around to help you this chapter is for you. It will show you how to give yourself a soothing Indian head massage, leaving you re-energized, calm and focused, easing your aching muscles and helping you to have a restful night's sleep. Get into the habit of giving yourself a massage at least once a week. You will find that it keeps stress at bay and replenishes vitality, leaving you refreshed and renewed. These simple yet effective techniques will help you to help yourself wherever and whenever you choose.

# Using Oils

We have already seen how oil can often be incorporated into Indian head massage. Indeed, Indian women often use oil to keep their hair lustrous and strong. Oil applied to the head is absorbed into the roots of the hair, strengthening it and removing dryness, which is responsible for brittle hair and for some scalp disorders. Oil can soften the skin of the scalp, promote hair growth, slow down hair loss and create vibrant, shiny hair. Regular self massage using oil is an effective way of keeping your hair in tip top condition.

As the oils are partially absorbed through the pores of the skin, the best ones to use are pure organic oils. Their effect is both internal and external. I personally recommend:

Sesame      Mustard      Almond      Coconut

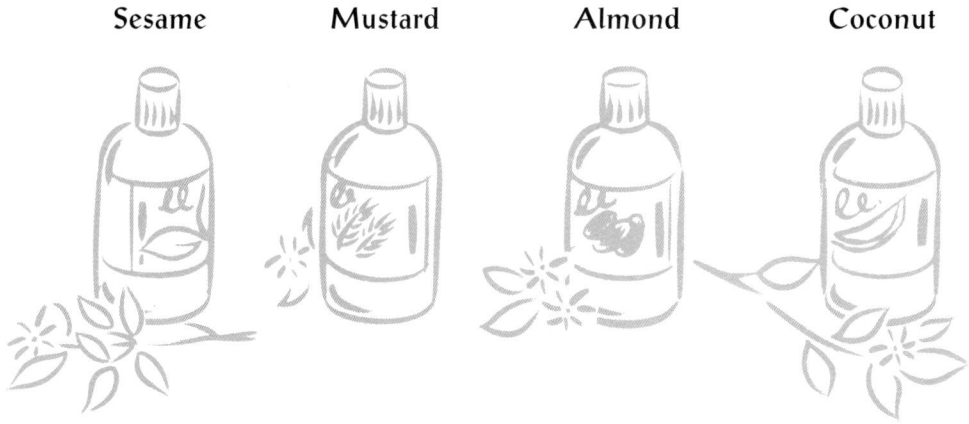

## SESAME OIL

This is probably the most popular oil in India. It is highly recommended within Ayurvedic medicine and Indian Champissage. Sesame oil is the best general oil. It reduces swelling, relieves muscular pains, stiffness, and strengthens and moisturizes the skin. Furthermore, because this oil contains iron and phosphorous, it is particularly recommended in Ayurveda. It is believed to keep hair in healthy condition and to be effective in delaying greying of the hair. It is also recommended for general body massage. It is a good balancing oil, and is traditionally used in the summer. It may irritate sensitive skin: if this happens, use olive oil instead.

## MUSTARD OIL

Mustard oil is one of the most popular oils in Northern India. This pungent oil gives a warming sensation. It is effective in increasing body heat and relieving pains, swelling and stiff muscles. It helps to cleanse the blood by opening the pores and it has a general strengthening and moisturizing effect. Since this oil creates a sensation of heat, it is particularly recommended for use during the winter.

## OLIVE OIL

This is freely available in the West and, in addition to being a good cooking oil, it can be applied to the body to relieve muscular stiffness and pain, increase body heat and reduce swelling. This is a good oil to use in the summer and is a suitable alternative to sesame oil.

## ALMOND OIL

This is a popular massage oil in the West and is good for warming the body and reducing any pain or stiffness. Suitable for both men and women, this oil can be used freely to help promote healthy hair.

## COCONUT OIL

This oil may be a little difficult to find in the West, but it is worth the effort since it has a beautiful aroma and is a pleasure to work with. Traditionally used in the spring, coconut oil is a light oil which can help to moisturize the skin, encourage healthy hair growth and balance the body in the process. As coconut oil is solid at room temperature, liquify it by standing it in warm water for a few minutes before use.

# PREPARING YOURSELF FOR MASSAGE

You can carry out self massage anywhere, but it is best to try and find somewhere quiet where you can be alone and concentrate on the healing power of your fingers. Make sure the room you choose is warm enough.

Sit with both feet on the ground, shoulders back, eyes closed, hands in your lap. Concentrate on your breathing. Try breathing deeply in and out through your nose and repeat this three times. Feel your ribcage expand and imagine your everyday worries are being expelled with each breath. Keeping your eyes closed, try and visualize yourself in a warm, sunny garden. Imagine the warmth of the sun melting away the stiffness in your muscles. Then concentrate on each body part in turn. Feel your arms and hands: can you feel any pain? Imagine the pain is seeping out of your muscles and your arms are feeling heavy and warm. Next, concentrate on your shoulders: imagine the pain disappearing, leaving your shoulders smooth and flexible. Now concentrate on your head: look up and down and side to side, imagine that the stiffness is draining away, leaving the muscles warm and relaxed. Visualize your face muscles becoming soft and smooth. Try to smile and hold the smile for a few seconds. Repeat the whole sequence.

Feel that your whole body is warm and the day's tension is melting away. Concentrate again on your breathing. When you are ready, open your eyes. Stretch your arms out to the sides and then take them up above your head. Stretch your body up.

Now you are ready to begin your self massage.

# YOUR STEP-BY-STEP GUIDE

Follow these simple steps to experience the beauty of a head massage just for one.

1 Pour some oil into your hand and apply it to the top of the head (on the crown).

2 Pour some more oil into your hand, and rub it between both palms. Massage the oil into your head, starting from the sides and working towards the top. Next, work your way towards the front and the back of the head, thus covering your entire head. This will distribute the oil evenly.

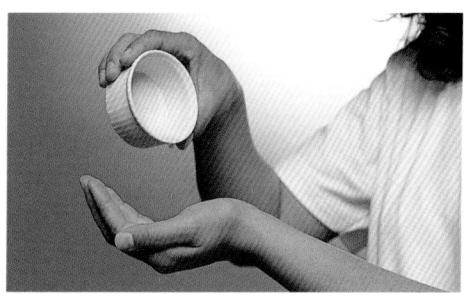

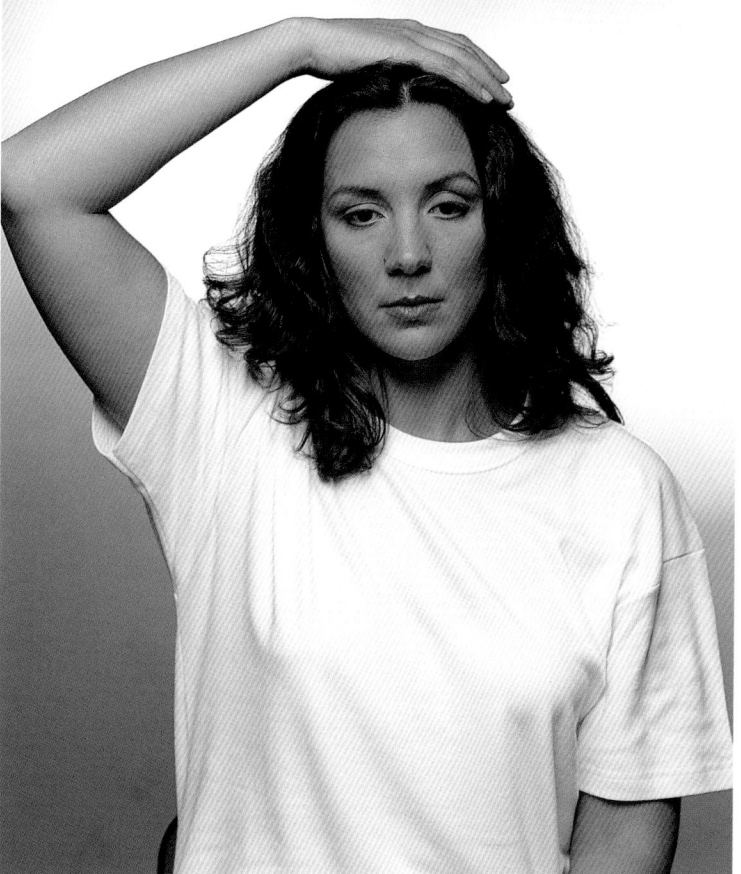

## SOLO MASSAGE

• I prefer to use oil with this self massage, but it can still be an effective destressor without it.

• Wear something loose and comfortable that allows you to move your arms about freely.

• If you are using oil choose clothes that won't be ruined if the oil gets onto them.

• If possible, shut the door, make sure you won't be disturbed and enjoy having this special time to yourself.

3 Now gently massage the whole of the area with your thumbs and fingers, releasing any tension by friction and rubbing.

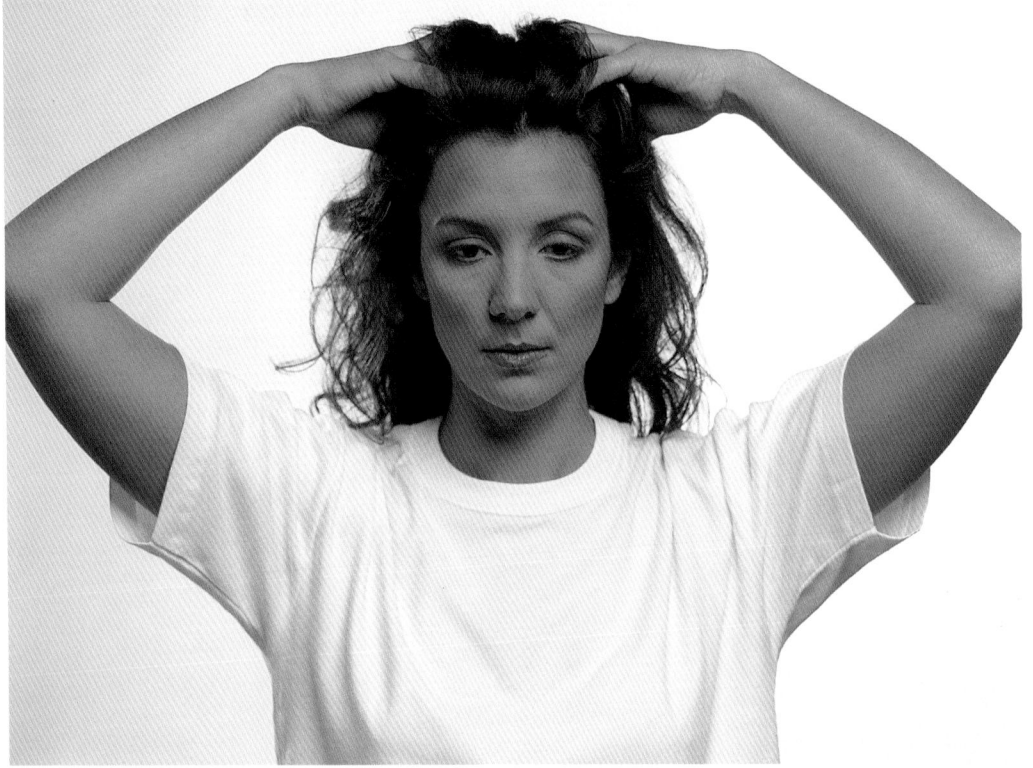

'The techniques are an invaluable treatment for the stress-linked troubles of modern life.' Gibraltar Chronicle

**TIME TO THINK**

In our hectic modern world it can be difficult to find time to spend on ourselves, particularly if we share our living space with others. Making time for regular self massage can give us the time we need to be still and listen to our own inner voice.

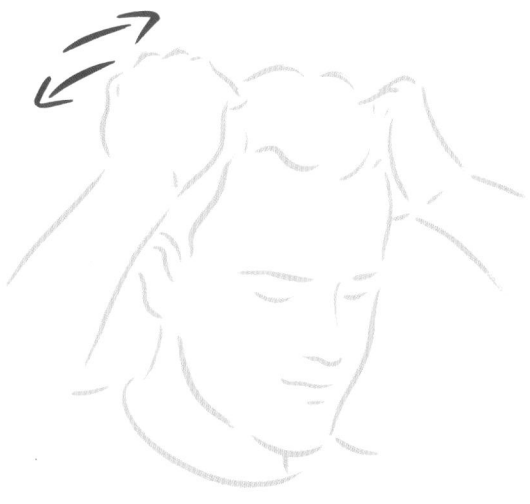

**4** Grasp fistfuls of hair at the roots and tug from side to side, keeping your knuckles very close to the scalp.

'The focus is on nourishing the person and encouraging self contact.' Rainbow Ark

**5** Squeeze at the temples with the heels of the hands and make slow, wide circular movements.

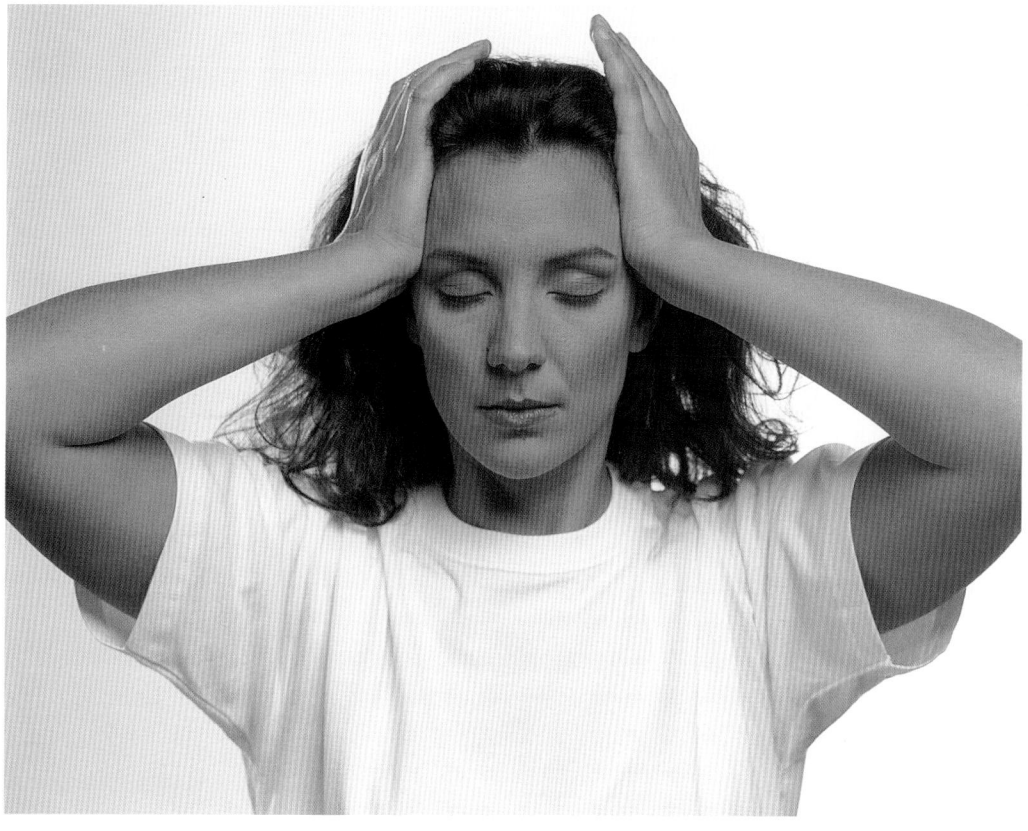

**6** Look down slightly and massage the back of the neck by squeezing and rolling the muscles. Start at the top of the neck and work your way down, first with one hand and then with the other hand. Repeat this a few times.

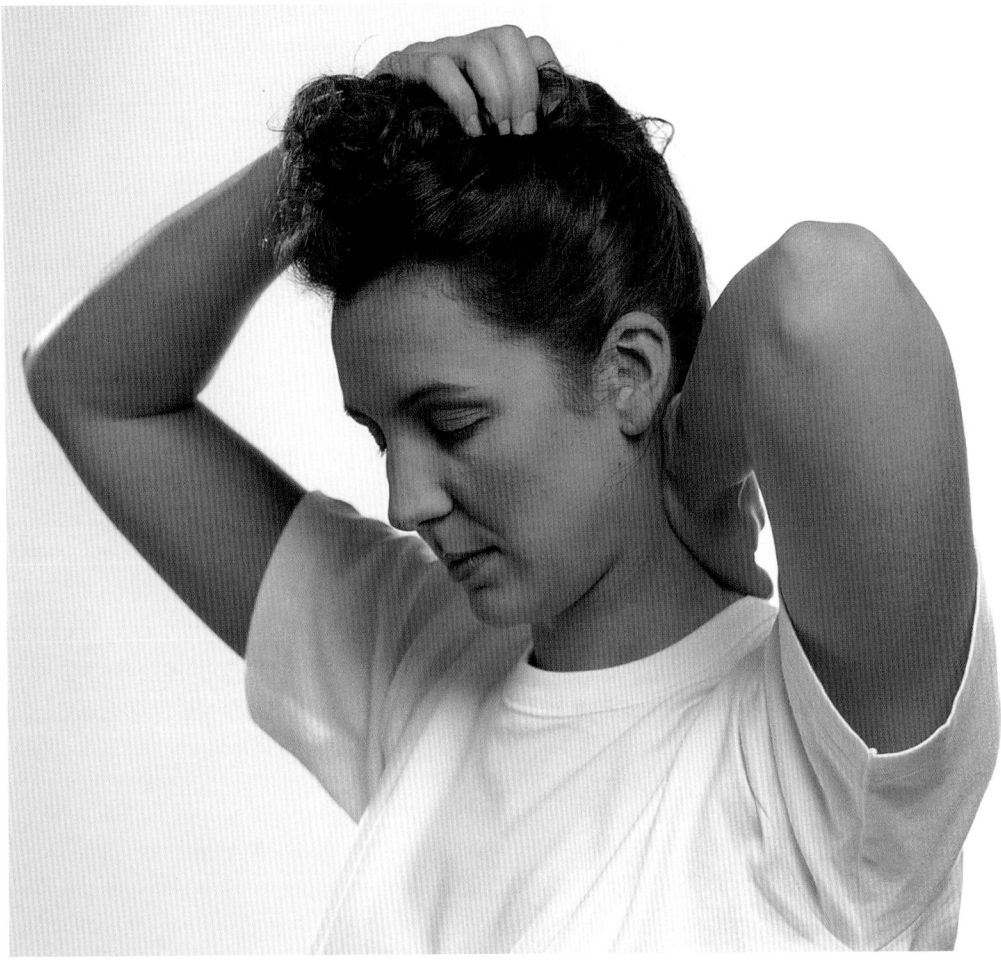

## NECK STRAIN

The back of our neck contains a complex network of muscles and nerves and so is particularly vulnerable to tension and strains. The techniques shown here are excellent for relieving stiff, sore neck muscles and minor strains.

*'A firm rub about the skull to relieve tension and a soothing stroke on the top of it to lift depression: sheer ecstasy.'* Good Housekeeping

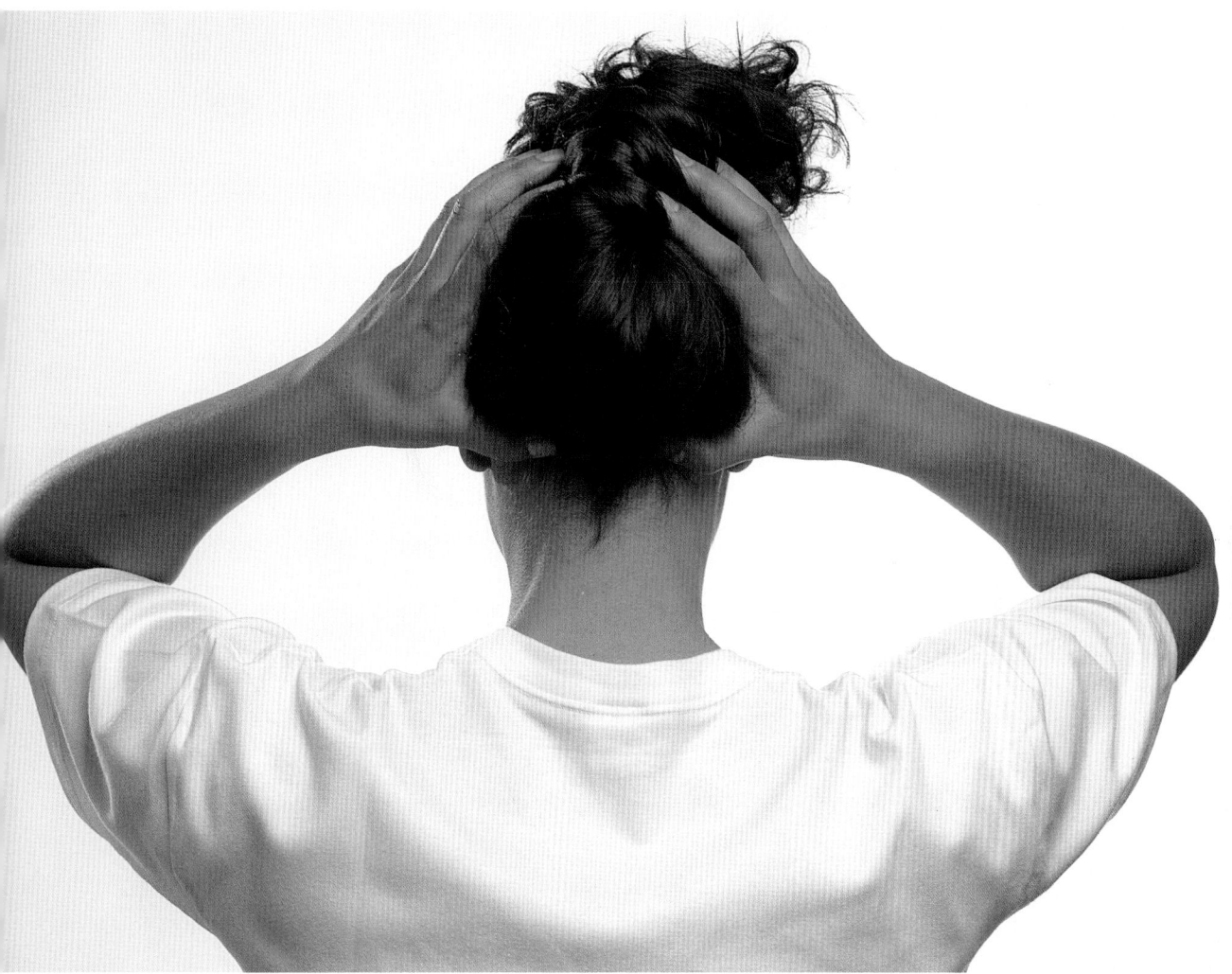

**7** Place the thumb of your left hand under the left occipital area and the thumb of your right hand under the right occipital area (base of the head) and relax the tight muscles by using friction or a rubbing movement.

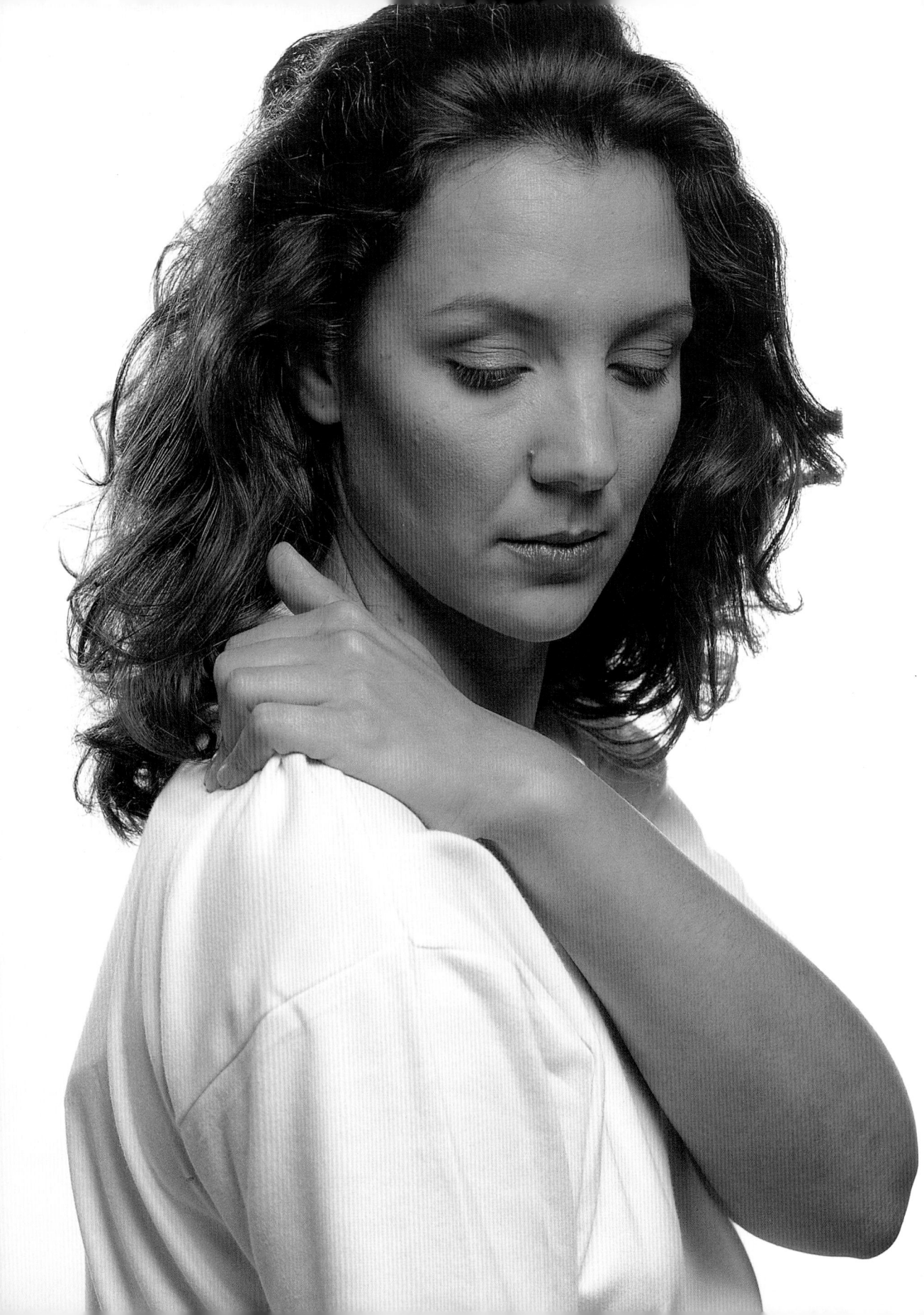

**8** Place your right hand on your left shoulder near your neck. Using medium pressure, gently squeeze the shoulder muscle that starts at the base of your neck.

Work your way outwards along your shoulder to your arm and then down as far as your elbow. When you reach your elbow, go back to the base of your neck and do this twice more. Concentrate on squeezing the muscle tissue.

This squeezing technique will improve blood circulation and help to release and disperse toxins from tight muscles. You can help the removal of toxins from your body by drinking plenty of water.

# Love yourself with a head massage just for one

**9** Now, place the flattened palm of your right hand beside the base of your neck on the left-hand side. Rub along the top of your left shoulder and continue down your left arm where you squeezed the muscles before. When you reach your elbow, go back to the base of the neck and repeat the action twice. Change arms and work the other side. This rubbing technique will help to release and disperse toxins from tight muscles and improve blood circulation. You can help in the removal of toxins by drinking plenty of mineral water.

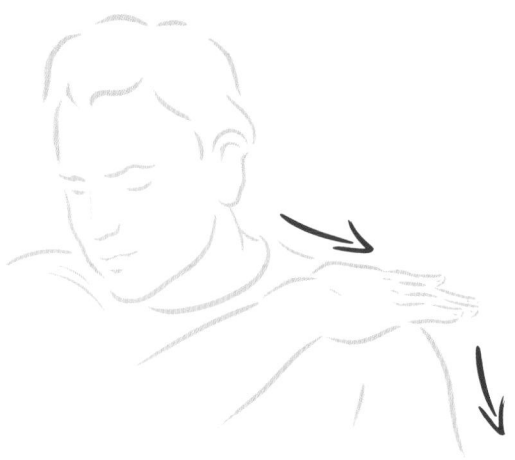

**10** Finally, rub lightly with your hands all over the head. Extend this movement to cover your face.

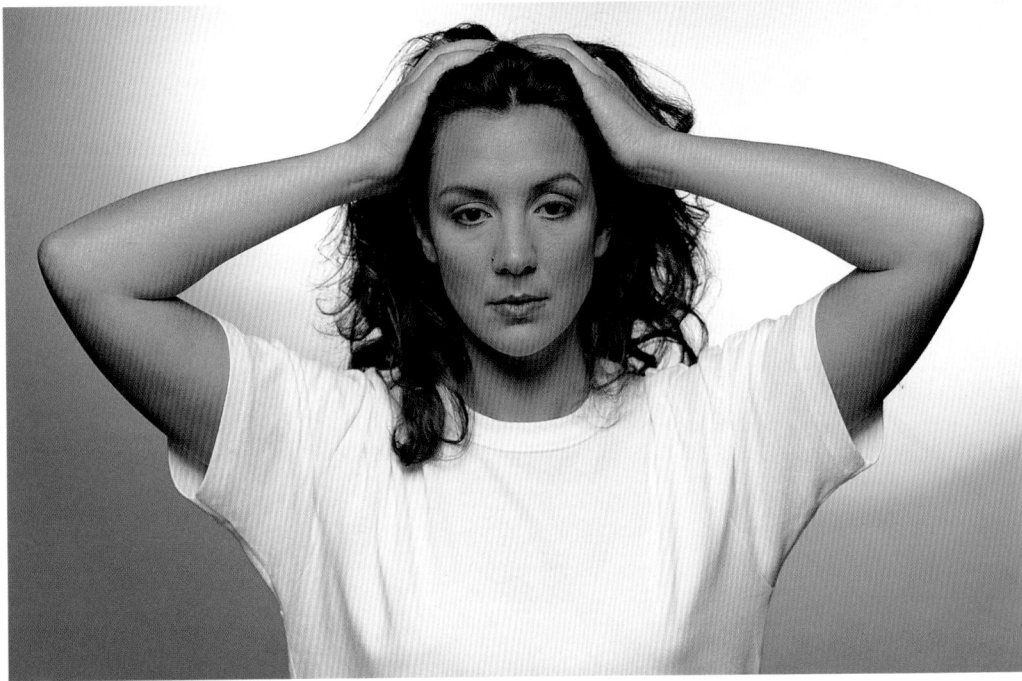

This self-massage will induce total relaxation. Don't forget you can use these movements anywhere, at any time, without the use of oil. If possible, always allow a few minutes after a massage session to relax your body and mind or carry out a few gentle stretching exercises.

# NECK STRETCHES

These exercises are designed to be done after the self-massage or anytime you feel tension in your neck. Do not attempt these exercises if you are suffering from any kind of neck injury.

Each exercise should be held for a count of four and repeated three times.

1   Stretch your neck by looking up and pointing your chin towards the ceiling. As you look up as far as you can, breathe in and hold the extended position. Breathe out and return to the previous position.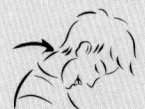

2   Breathe in, then as you are breathing out, look down as far as possible with your chin almost touching your chest. Then breathe in again, returning to the previous position.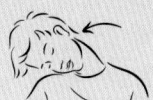

3   Begin with your head in the upright position. Breathe in and then bend your neck towards the right so that your right ear is almost touching your right shoulder. Keep your shoulders down. Breathe out and return your head to the upright position.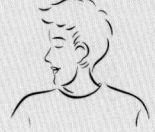

4   Repeat exercise 3, bending your neck to the left-hand side.

5   Begin with your head in the upright position. Breathe in and look over your right shoulder as far as possible. Then breathe out and return.

6   Repeat exercise 5, looking over your left shoulder.

These exercises are wonderful for relieving stiffness and tension in the neck muscles. They loosen up the muscles and increase neck mobility. If your neck is relaxed and supple, the blood flow to your brain increases, improving your concentration and ability to think clearly. Remember to be gentle: don't stretch too far.

Everyone needs and can benefit from massage, whether it is self massage, massage given by a friend or a professional therapist. However, you should try to have a massage from a professional therapist from time to time to get the most benefit.

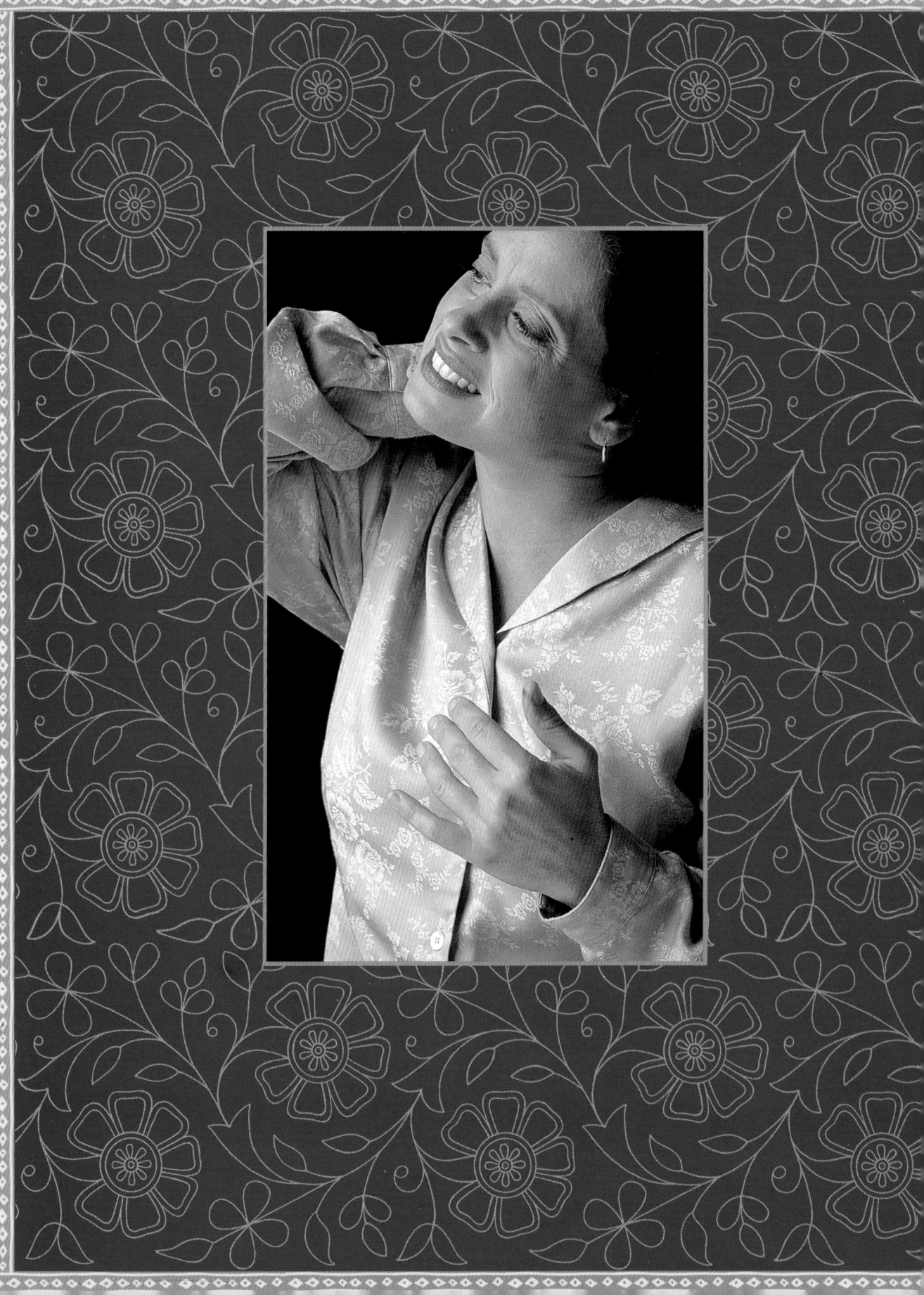

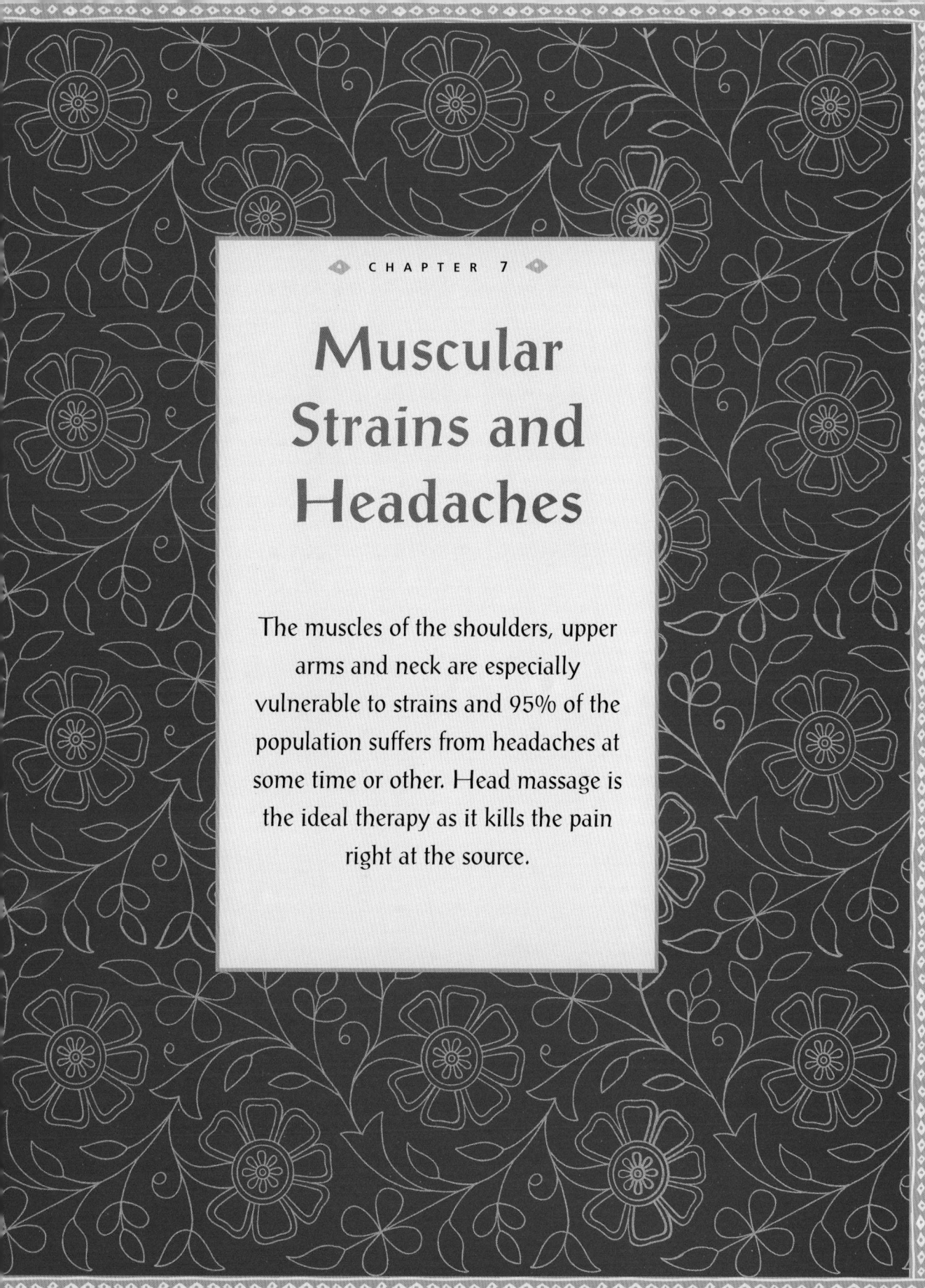

# CHAPTER 7

# Muscular Strains and Headaches

The muscles of the shoulders, upper arms and neck are especially vulnerable to strains and 95% of the population suffers from headaches at some time or other. Head massage is the ideal therapy as it kills the pain right at the source.

# INTRODUCTION

The human body is an extremely complex organism, comprised of a combination of elements: physical, emotional, intellectual and spiritual. Each of these elements is designed to work in perfect unison with every other. The four components are all interlinked and essential to the whole, and each one reacts with the others, creating either harmony or disturbance. Each element needs to be kept in balance to maintain the body's equilibrium. So it follows that any emotional problem, such as unexpressed anxiety or anger, may result in physical strain, pain or illness, while an over reliance on the intellect, leading to excessive anxiety, overwork and lack of exercise, can result in emotional stress and tension in the muscles. It is common to find that emotional problems manifest themselves in the upper back, shoulders, neck and head, and this area is therefore prone to strains, injuries, illness and distortion of the muscles in the body and face. Work on these areas through Indian head massage can release built-up tension from the muscles, relieving a variety of symptoms over time, and helping to rebalance and realign the body. This brings about a feeling of mental and emotional, as well as physical, well-being.

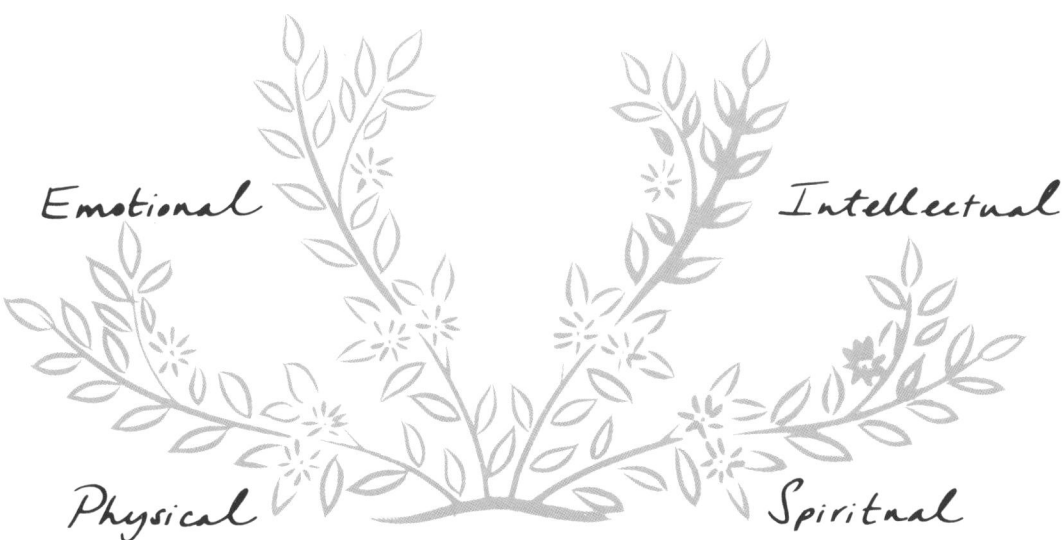

Emotional          Intellectual

Physical          Spiritual

# How Muscles Work

The muscles are a collection of specialized cells that have the ability to change their length and breadth by easy and rapid expansion and contraction. Muscle can be stimulated to contract to such an extent that it moves bones. The stimulation to move muscles is either voluntary, that is, it is under the control of the will, or involuntary and without any direct control from the individual. We all exercise our voluntary muscles every time we move around, pick something up or turn our head, while involuntary muscles regulate our body's functions: our heartbeats and our breathing.

The muscles that we use to move around have an 'origin' and an 'insertion' point where they attach to the bone. The origin is a fixed point of attachment that does not move when the muscle contracts. The insertion point, however, can move with the bone.

# Easing Muscle Strain or Injury

Muscles can easily be damaged by being overstretched, torn or bruised. When this happens, the muscle frequently goes into spasm. This is the body's primitive, but effective, way of preventing us from moving the muscle and damaging it further. However, the muscle spasm restricts the flow of blood to the damaged area and so hinders the healing process. To repair muscle damage and restore the functioning of each damaged part, the muscle spasm must first be relaxed. Indian head massage does just that.

## The Neck

Muscular strain and spasm in the neck muscles is a common condition. It is often a result of a sports injury but can also be caused by sleeping with insufficient neck and head support, especially where there is a history of neck injury. Pain can either come on suddenly, after a particular movement, or gradually, over time.

A muscle spasm may either hold the head in a 'tilted to one side' position or manifest itself in pain in the side of the neck or in any of the muscles in that area, for example, the levator scapulae, rhomboideus major, sterno-cleido-mastoid, scalenus, splenius capitis or the trapezius. Pain and stiffness in the neck may also be caused by inflammation of the soft tissue through a build-up of urea and lactic acid, a condition known as

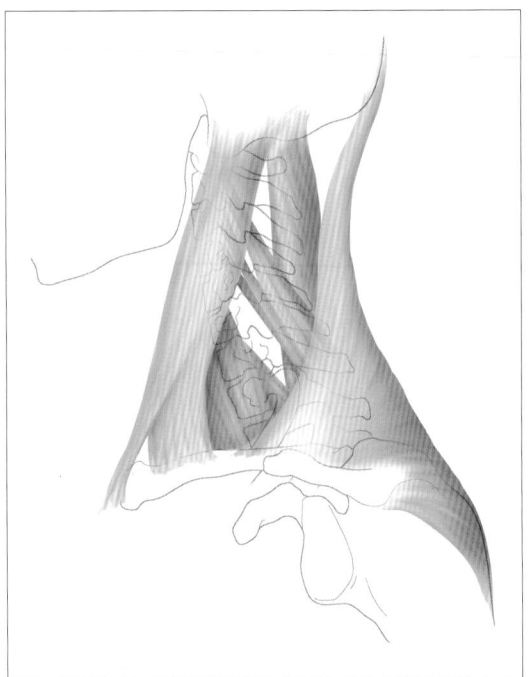

fibrositis. Torticollis, or wry neck, is due to the inflammation of the sterno-cleido-mastoid muscle. The inflammation results in muscle contraction, leaving the sufferer with their neck bent over to one side. There are several factors that contribute to the inflammation, but it is thought that damp weather and a sudden change in temperature can aggravate it.

Indian head massage includes various techniques for use on these muscles, in particular the friction movement along the neck muscles. Friction and rubbing underneath the occipital area (base of the head) and the grasp and pull back technique are also very beneficial. Gentle neck exercises are recommended along with localized heat treatment.

Other conditions of the neck and spine that can benefit from regular Indian head massage include: cervical spondylosis (a degenerative change in the intervertebral discs) which tends to affect people over 50 and produces pain and stiffness in the neck which can spread to the shoulders and arms; and cervical spondylitis (inflammation of the vertebrae of the spine), a condition that can lead to ankylosing spondylitis, or poker spine.

## The Shoulders

The shoulder area is one of the most common areas of tension. Stiffening and loss of flexibility of the upper back and shoulders may have many causes, ranging from muscle strain, emotional tension and bad posture to repetitive movement. These problems and others can have a restrictive effect on the ribs, breathing and, circulation, eventually throwing the whole body out of balance. Weakened or strained muscles in the shoulder area can lead to a wide range of problems that can have a significant effect on the sufferer's life. A weakened upper trapezius can result in an inability to raise the arms to the sides or above the head, and can cause the shoulder on the affected side to end up lower than the other. Stiffness or tightness in the rhomboids results in aching and soreness between the shoulder blades that can feel like a tightened rope, while a weakness of the serratus anterior muscle leads to difficulty in pushing the arms straight out in front. A strained supraspinatus muscle, caused by long hours in intense concentration at a desk or in a car, or by shoulder dislocation, will create difficulty in moving the arm away from the body.

Stiffness or strain in the levator scapulae can affect mobility of the neck in rotation and side-bending.

Indian head massage includes a very effective programme for treatment of the shoulder and upper arm. The programme not only relaxes the muscles but also stimulates the blood and lymphatic system to help eliminate toxins and speed the healing of damaged muscles. Movement of the shoulder can often be regained with the help of specific shoulder mobilization techniques carried out by a

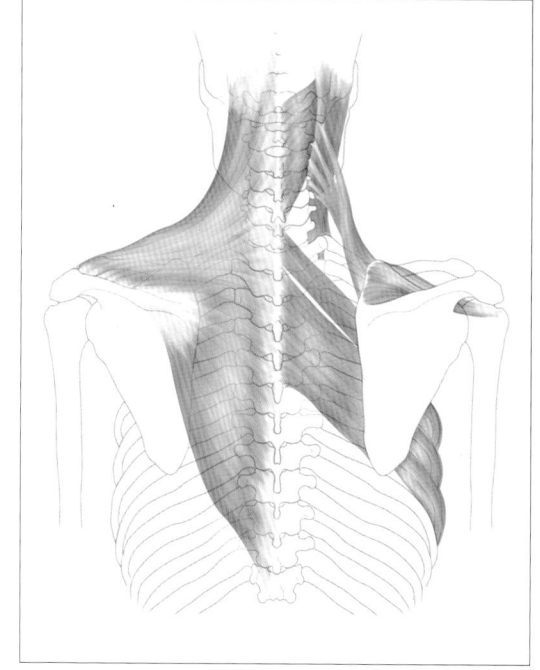

qualified practitioner, along with lots of mid-back friction and other upper back techniques. Very often, when there is a tightness in the muscles of the upper back and around the shoulder, pain is felt in the arms, and so some time should be spent on these. Once all the surrounding muscles have been warmed, gentle shoulder rotation should then be carried out. Gentle shoulder lifts can be tried with caution. The client is recommended to sit straight with shoulders back as often as possible in the day to correct the posture.

### TENDON INJURIES IN THE SHOULDER

The shoulder joint is supported by a group of small muscles and tendons called the rotator cuff. Four short tendons hold the upper end of the arm bone (humerus) in the shoulder socket. Sudden forceful injuries can cause a small tear, or even a rupture of one of these tendons. Excessive, repetitive movements, such as swimming, racket sports, weight lifting and computer work can cause swelling and inflammation of one of these tendons (tendonitis). The swollen tendon then gets 'pinched' between the shoulder bone and the humerus during certain movements (usually on raising the arm out to one side.) Injury can be 'acute', because of a tear, or chronic, due to overuse. An acute injury needs gentle and specialist treatment, whereas chronic pain from overuse simply needs rest.

Gentle mobilizing movements are important to maintain general mobility and all the Indian head massage techniques which cover the shoulders, arms and neck are recommended. Rubbing, hacking, squeezing and friction across the muscle fibres will all increase blood circulation and help to heal, although these would not be recommended directly over the site of an acute injury.

# ROUNDED OR RAISED SHOULDERS, CONCAVE CHESTS AND IMPAIRED BREATHING

These conditions can develop over many years for a variety of reasons. A person's lifestyle, his or her negative attitudes, a depressive character or even anxiety about body size and shape can all lead to physical deformities: embarrassment about large breasts or being too tall can both cause stooping and hunching. Permanent stress or tension can result in raised shoulders: a habit which forms in early life and becomes a permanent problem later on.

Lots of friction and massage in the trapezius/rhomboids, combined with regular shoulder mobilization techniques and strong pressure to the sides of the spine to ease the shoulders back into a more natural position is recomended, and encouragement to sit up with a more lifted spine may help a person's awareness of correct posture. Asking someone to imagine a string attached to the top of their head, pulling them up towards the ceiling, can help to correct posture. Regular Indian head massage can also help to bring about a different mental state – it helps a person feel more able to cope with life's stress through the development of relaxation. The advanced form of head massage – Champissage – can help to balance energy, allowing a person to feel more confident and centred. These positive changes in mental attitude can often bring dramatic physical changes in their wake.

Impaired breathing may also be improved by the same head massage techniques and breathing problems can often be corrected by learning and practising deep abdominal and yogic breathing.

# EYE STRAIN

Most of us take it for granted that we are able to focus with ease on objects at a great variety of distances: from a book just in front of our face to a distant mountain on the horizon. We are unaware of the processes that take place within our eyes to enable this to happen. The ability to focus is controlled by the ciliary muscles, which relax and contract to accommodate the need for different lengths of focus.

When the eye is at rest, the ciliary muscles are in a relaxed state and the eye naturally focuses on distant objects. In order for the eye to focus on closer objects, the ciliary muscles must contract. The ciliary muscles are therefore working very hard if a great amount of close work is done, and this results in eyestrain.

The following situations will cause or exacerbate eyestrain:

◆ Watching television for long periods

◆ Reading for long periods in poor light

◆ Age: the ability of the muscles to focus well deteriorates as a person gets older

◆ Stress, as this causes the muscles of the head and face to tighten

◆ Wearing old glasses or not wearing glasses when they are needed

Time spent during an Indian head massage treatment on the squeeze and lift and circular temple friction techniques (see pages 62 and 65) will help, as will scalp massage and hair tugging. These techniques, combined with the application of pressure on the ridge of the bone all around the eyes at least twice, relax the muscles and give immediate relief. For those who suffer from persistent eye strain a visit to an optician is recommended to ensure that any visual problems are correctly treated.

## CASE HISTORY

Age: 38
Sex: Male
Profession: Long distance lorry driver

◆ Symptoms: David complained of sore muscles in the shoulders and upper arms and very restricted movement in the neck. He felt exhausted at the end of every day.
◆ After the first treatment: He almost nodded off.
◆ After the third treatment: David reported lessening of pain in the shoulders but said that his upper arms were still aching.
◆ After subsequent treatments: He was pleased that he could move his neck further than before without any pain. He felt more energetic, which he thought was due to better quality sleep. He looked forward to each treatment and couldnÕt imagine life without Indian head massage.
◆ Further recommendations: I suggested that he should try to have regular treatments, or come whenever he could.

## CASE HISTORY

Age: 35
Sex: Male
Profession: Manual worker

◆ Symptoms: Peter has a chronic whiplash injury, caused by a driving accident a few years back. He had never tried massage as he had been wrongly advised that it could make his condition worse. However, he was currently experiencing severe pain in the neck and shoulder and was encouraged by his wife, one my clients, to come to me for help.
◆ After the first treatment: Peter felt relaxed and sleepy.
◆ After the third treatment: Peter was delighted at the increased range of movement in his neck and that his tight muscles were becoming softer. I spent a large portion of each treatment working on the muscles of his neck and shoulders.
◆ After subsequent treatments: Peter was very pleased to find that he could take his head back much further than before without any discomfort. He felt as though a great weight had been lifted from his shoulders.
◆ Further recommendations: I suggested that Peter continue with regular sessions to improve his condition.

## HEADACHES

The brain itself and most of the brain covering cannot feel any pain, but the blood vessels in the brain are interlaced with many nerves. These nerves are especially sensitive to changes of blood pressure within the skull, and it is in these nerves that the pain of a headache originates. Many conditions can cause a pressure change within the skull, and trigger a headache.

Most recurrent headaches are due to tension or migraine. Sometimes the origin of a headache can be traced to other parts of the body, and certain conditions are known to trigger headaches:

- ◆ Eyestrain
- ◆ Sinusitis
- ◆ Influenza
- ◆ Hay fever
- ◆ Menstruation
- ◆ High blood pressure
- ◆ Hunger
- ◆ Lack of sleep
- ◆ Excessive alcohol consumption
- ◆ A noisy environment

Such headaches can only be treated effectively by getting at the cause. If a headache is accompanied by nausea, fever, vomiting or disturbed vision professional advice should be sought.

# TENSION HEADACHES

Around 40–50% of all headaches fall into the category of tension headaches. The basic cause of a tension headache is the contraction of muscles over the scalp, forehead, back of head, upper part of the neck and around the jaw. Tension headaches characteristically occur at midday or in the afternoon and evening. They may be brief or they may last several hours or days. The severity varies. Sometimes the pain will be of low intensity but persistent. It can be boring, sharp, bursting or exploding and it is commonly experienced as a feeling of a tight band around the head. The head may feel as if it is being compressed or squeezed in a vice. Tension headaches can occur without any other symptoms and are believed to be due mainly to emotional stress.

An overload of stress can make a person extremely tired yet unable to sleep or relax sufficiently to cope with the stress. Just what constitutes an 'overload' of stress is difficult to describe – some people seem to cope more easily with stressful situations than others. However, it is common to find people suffering from stress-related headaches in our modern age. Stressful situations set up a process of knotting the muscles in the shoulders and neck, and they begin to ache and cause pain. The person then complains

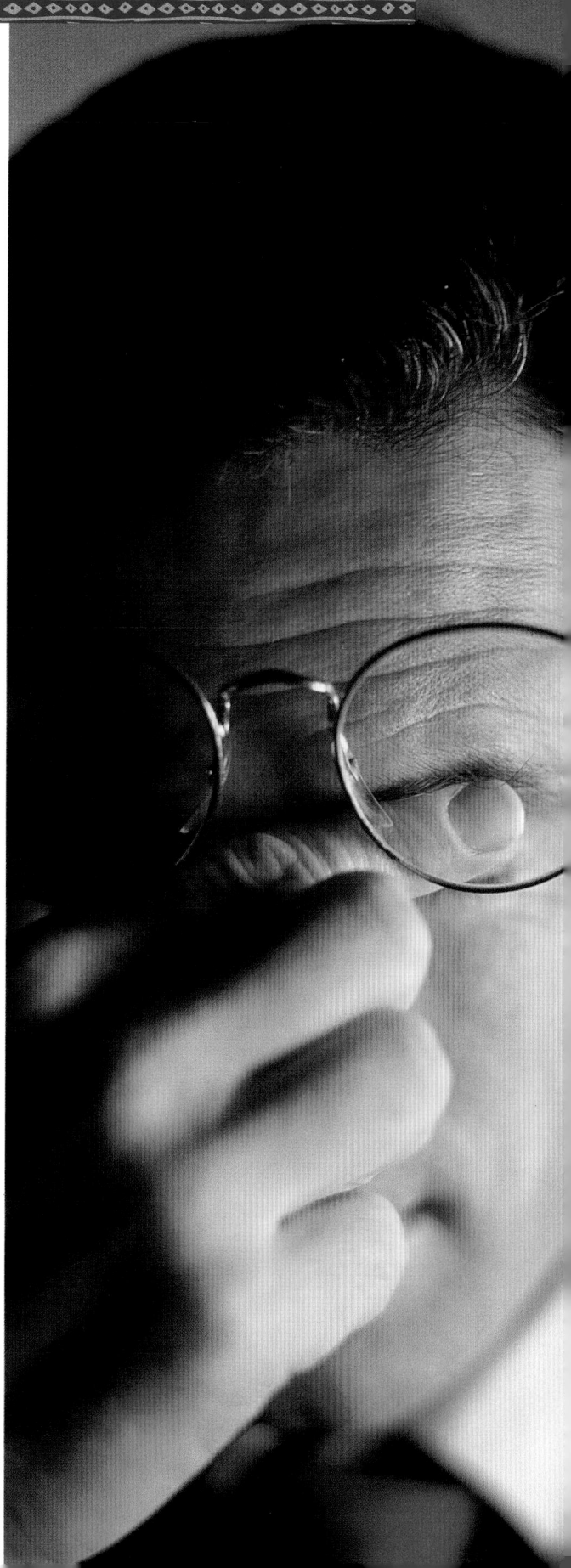

of pain thumping around inside the head, or experiences painful areas in and around the head, neck and shoulders.

This type of headache can often be relieved immediately by Indian head massage. A combination of neck and head massage techniques with friction applied across the tender, ropy muscles in the neck and across the base of the skull will begin to ease the pain. Scalp massage techniques including friction, rubbing the base of the scalp and slow circular head movements will also contribute to the easing of tension headaches.

Indian head massage encourages relaxation and lowers stress and so treats the cause of the headache. In addition, people who suffer from tension headaches may be able to identify and avoid the stressor that causes the headache in the first place.

'A skilful massage is an excellent way of relieving stresses... headaches and eyestrain.'

Manchester Evening News

# MIGRAINE

Like tension headaches, these cannot usually be traced to any general bodily disorder. An attack may come on without apparent cause, or it may follow some emotional disturbance. The basis of migraine is an excessive sensitivity of the blood vessels of the head. This sensitivity involves arteries and capillaries over the face and scalp and inside the skull. Attacks may last several hours. Typically, at the beginning of the attack the blood vessels narrow down and become constricted. As a result the blood supply to part of the head is reduced. A section of the brain, the eyes or the nerves are deprived of oxygen. The attack may begin with a warning phase consisting of blurred vision, numbness, or other sensations depending upon which part of the head is temporarily short of blood and oxygen. As the constriction wears off, the headache begins to develop. The blood vessels widen and dilate and the distended vessels become pain-sensitive. Muscles may become tense and contract.

In migraine the disturbances can be quite complex and are not necessarily limited to the head. Thus there may be:

◆ Changes in mood with feelings of well-being just before the attacks start and later irritation, depression and even aggression.

◆ Changes in sleep and wakefulness. Before the attack one may feel sleepy and start yawning as the attack commences. Afterwards people often feel more awake.

◆ Changes in appetite. It is not unusual to feel ravenously hungry before attacks and quite unable to eat during the actual attack.

◆ Increased sensitivity to smells and noises during an attack.

Age: 39
Sex: Female
Profession: Office manager

◆ Symptoms: This office manager came to my clinic complaining bitterly about her migraines. Carol works in a busy office and has lots of responsibilities. To make matters worse, Carol also suffers from disturbed sleep. Her first visit coincided with a migraine attack.
◆ After the first treatment: Carol said her headache had gone. She felt as if an enormous weight had been lifted from her, and that as the pressure had dropped, so had her shoulders.
◆ After subsequent treatments: After six treatments, she had only one migraine attack, which lasted just one instead of the usual three days. Carol was pleased she was sleeping much better. She woke up every morning feeling full of energy.
◆ Further recommendations: Regular head massages as she works in a stressful environment.

Migraine, is an intermittent, often one-sided headache with freedom from pain between attacks. The symptoms last anything from a day to several days and are often accompanied by visual or stomach disturbances. Migraine can often be provoked by stress, and dietary habits have also been implicated. Other characteristics of migraine include:

◆ A particularly devastating headache may come after a long, pain-free interval. Fourteen per cent of women subject to migraine have a definite tendency to have attacks before periods (pre-menstrual migraine).

◆ There may be a cyclical tendency. Thus some people have their attacks when under stress mid-week, and others as a let-down headache at the weekend.

◆ Disturbances in weight, sleep, mood, appetite, etc., may be related to attacks.

◆ There may be neurological symptoms such as numbness on one side of the face, pain in the upper jaw involving the teeth, blurred or partial loss of vision.

◆ At times there may be weakness or numbness down one half of the body occurring on the same side as the headache.

Migraines can usually be divided into three types:

### COMMON MIGRAINE

These are severe headaches that occur at regular intervals and usually affect only half the head. They are generally accompanied by eye disturbances and/or sickness. One in ten people are prone to common migraine.

### CLASSICAL MIGRAINE

This term applies to the type of severe, unilateral migraine that is preceded by warning signs, for example disturbed vision. The sufferer commonly sees zigzag patterns of light, brightly coloured spots or experiences islands of visual loss. These symptoms occur with the constriction of blood vessels and often last for 10 to 30 minutes before the onset of the headache. They are referred to as focal symptoms and relate anatomically to the blood vessels primarily involved. Less than one in 50 people are prone to this type of migraine.

### FOCAL MIGRAINE

Migraines known as focal migraines are even rarer than the classical migraine. In these, the symptoms of the migraine overshadow the actual headache attacks. The visual symptoms may be quite dramatic, with bright, scintillating, shimmering or coloured blobs causing patches of visual loss. Vision may be lost to one side, or both sides. The disturbances may appear hallucinatory with objects appearing larger, smaller, or as a mosaic, like broken coloured pebbles. Colours may be heightened or objects appear strange or unduly familiar. Double vision or drooping of the eyelid can occur.

During the course of a life-time, a person with migraine will find that the disorder may take several forms. In childhood the tendency may show as periodic vomiting, while in later age, as the tendency slowly wears off, other complaints, such as dizziness, occasionally replace the more usual headache. Relaxing in a warm bath followed by rest in bed may help to relieve a migraine headache. Indian head massage is often effective in easing the pain of a migraine attack. If you have an Indian head massage before an attack, or when one is suspected, then the attack may be delayed or the symptoms may be milder. I believe regular head massage will help you to extend the interval between the attacks, and in some cases the migraines may even disappear completely.

# Vascular Headaches

Vascular headaches arise from changes in the blood supply to the head. If there is an excess of red blood cells, the blood will be stickier and its flow reduced. If there are too few cells (as in anaemia) less oxygen will be carried to the brain. Both circumstances may result in painful headaches.

# Headaches Associated with Fever

About 10% of headaches are associated with fever. They occur mostly in the young and respond quickly to treatment. In women, a constant dull headache is often a symptom of cystitis. Headaches may be an early symptom of other infections such as food poisoning or 'flu and are also associated with viral illness, often persisting for weeks afterwards.

# Headaches Following Injury

Any injury to the head is likely to cause a headache, either immediately or later on. There may be tenderness at the site of the damage or a steady ache due to muscle spasm. Your head may throb, often on one side only, and you may experience some giddiness. A severe jolt to the neck may result in an ache that arises at the back of the neck and spreads forwards. Any of these types of pain may be worsened by noise, excitement, exertion, alcohol or head movement. In sport, repeated blows to the head may result in a migraine-like pain. If a headache is due to any of the causes described here, medical advice should be sought as soon as possible to rule out concussion or serious damage to the head. Head massage may not be appropriate in these cases.

# OTHER HEADACHES

## The Sinuses

The sinuses are four paired, air-filled cavities located in the skull near the nose. They are lined with mucous membrane and they help to warm and moisten the air we breathe. Pollution and large-scale consumption of dairy products sometimes causes the sinuses to become blocked or inflamed. A build up of fluid pressure can cause head and cheek pain.

## The Neck

Many pains arise from the neck due to contraction of muscles over the neck and scalp. This can be due to stress, bad posture or manual work. In older people it is commonly associated with arthritic changes. From around 50 years of age, neck movements generally become increasingly restricted and muscular head pains arising from the neck are more frequent. They may spread from the back of the head to behind the eyes or the temples.

## The Eyes

Many pains start around or behind the eyes but few, in practice, are related to eye disorders, although minor errors in refraction or squints may be to blame. Bad lighting conditions – too bright, too dim or flickering lights – especially at work – can induce head pain. In older people head pain may indicate the presence of pressure within the eye – glaucoma. The pain comes on gradually, is localized to the eye, but may then spread outwards and can be accompanied by nausea and vomiting.

## The Teeth and Jaw

The pain of migraine more often extends to the gums and teeth than toothache to the skull. Pains relating to muscles and joints of the lower jaw can cause widespread pain in the face and trigger off migraine attacks.

# RELIEVING THE PAIN

Indian head massage can be a great help in reducing headaches caused by tension, eye-strain and stiffness in the neck and shoulders. Sixty percent of all headaches are caused by these problems and Indian head massage is more effective than drugs because the cause is eliminated along with the symptoms. Painkilling drugs work simply by blocking the 'pain messages' sent to the brain, while head massage eradicates the pain messages by relaxing the constricted muscles that are causing the pain in the first place.

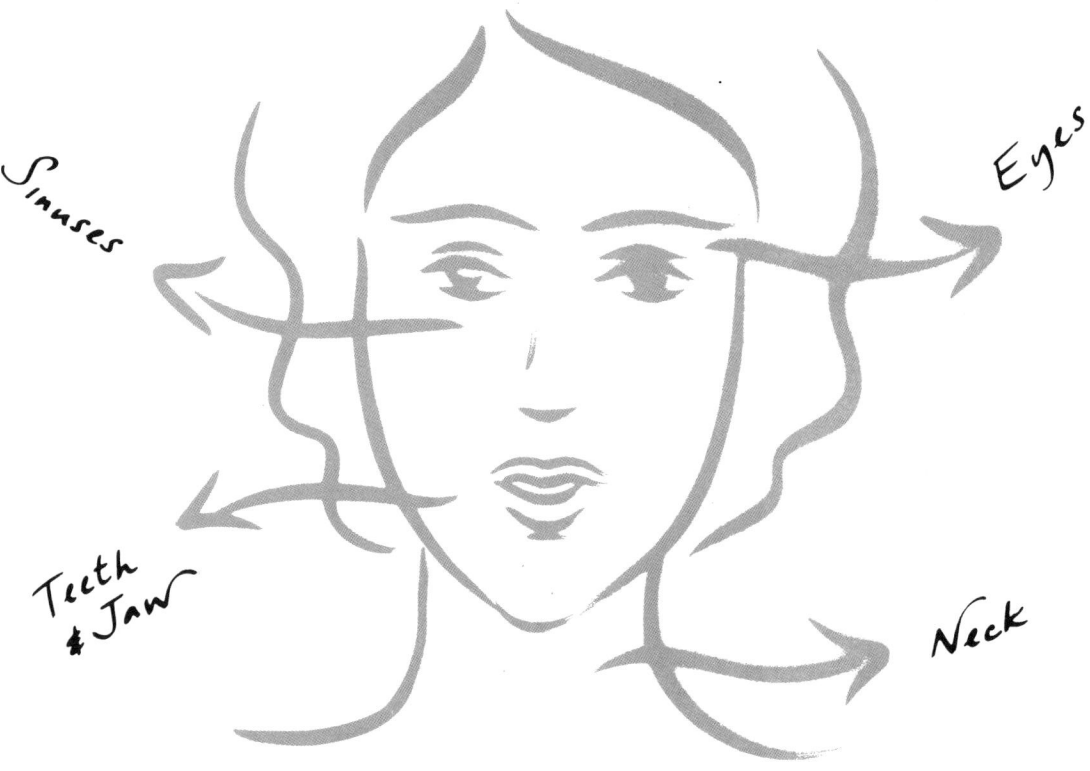

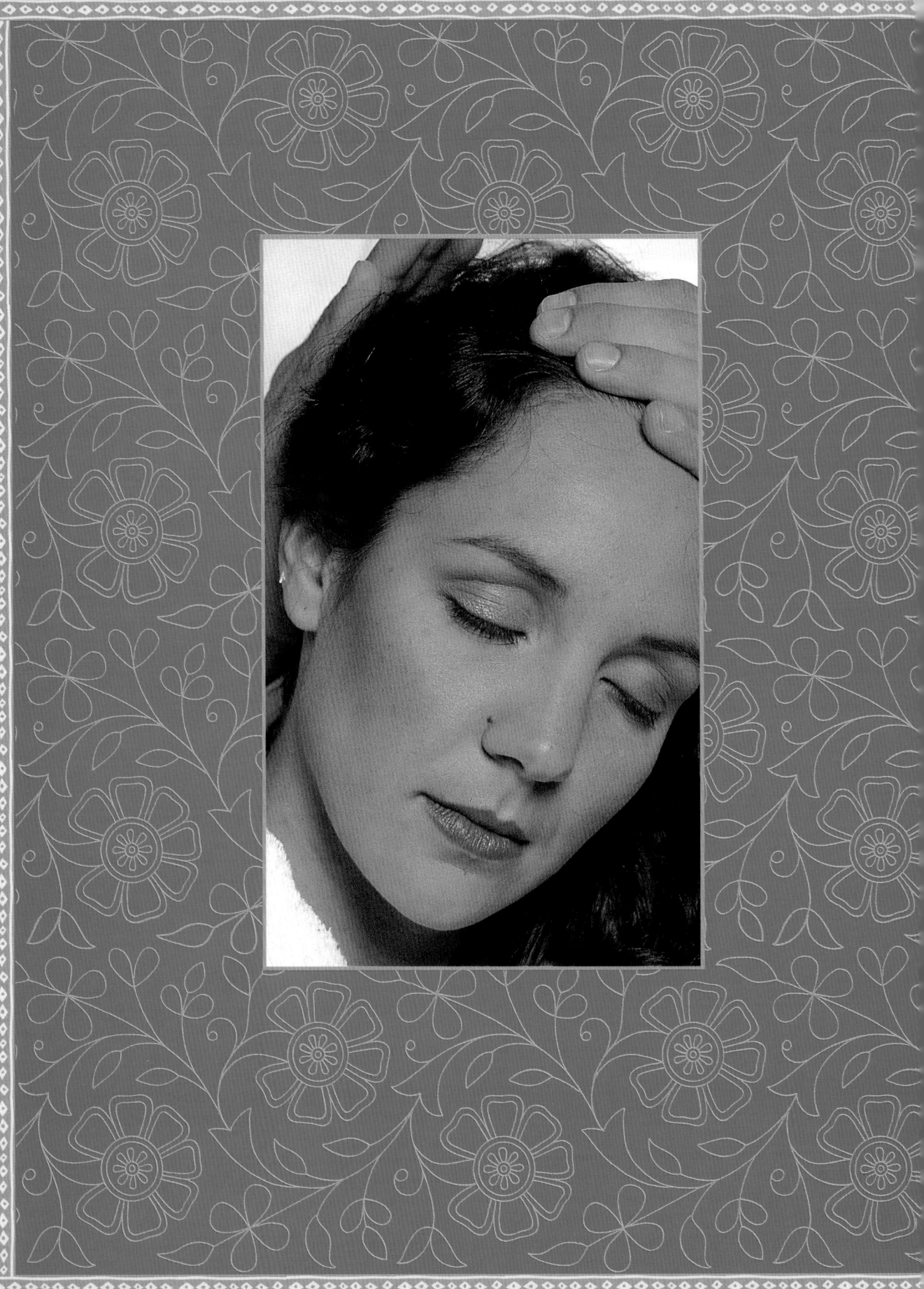

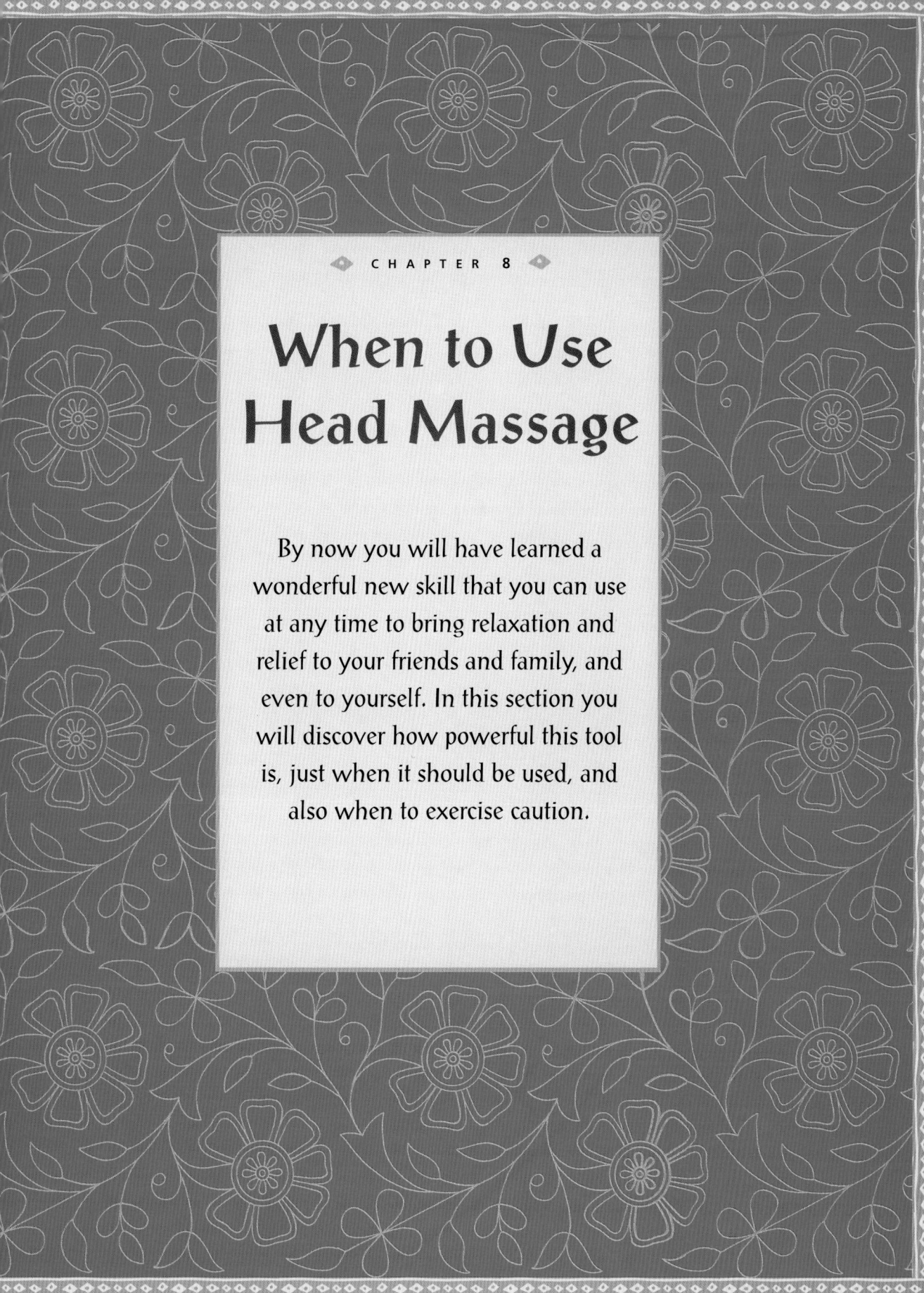

CHAPTER 8

# When to Use Head Massage

By now you will have learned a wonderful new skill that you can use at any time to bring relaxation and relief to your friends and family, and even to yourself. In this section you will discover how powerful this tool is, just when it should be used, and also when to exercise caution.

# INTRODUCTION

Indian head massage works on both a physical and a mental level. By concentrating on the areas most vulnerable to stress and tension, it provides a de-stressing programme for the whole body. Relieving tension in these key areas unlocks the energy trapped in the muscles, encouraging the flow of the blood and thereby re-energizing every part of the body. The results of freeing up this energy are felt on a mental, physical and spiritual level.

Indian head massage has a far-reaching effect on every one of the body's systems. It supports the nervous system by alleviating stress. By stimulating the lymphatic system, the process of eliminating toxins and poisons is encouraged, and our bodies are cleansed and purified more efficiently. The circulatory and immune systems are stimulated, and the respiratory system is reinforced, as deep breathing is encouraged.

The shoulder area acts as a buffer between the mind and the body, and attitudes to responsibilities, fear and suppressed feelings can all be reflected in this area of the body. Muscles tighten due to emotional and physical stress and the tight muscles impede the free movement of the neck and shoulders. Indian head massage helps by using a variety of stimulating and tension-releasing techniques. The stimulating strokes, such as champi, hacking and ironing down (see pages 43 and 82), help to increase the blood supply.

Massage of the upper arm helps to relax overused muscles, such as the biceps, triceps and deltoid. This helps to improve the mobility of the shoulder joint.

Massage of the face and scalp reduces the number of tension headaches and in some cases eliminates them. The most effective techniques in these areas are friction and rub under the occiput, whole hand friction and squeeze and lift on the scalp (see pages 51, 52, 58 and 62).

# PHYSICAL AND MENTAL BENEFITS

Here I have tried to provide a list of the physical and mental benefits of Indian head massage for your easy reference, but it is by no means an exhaustive list: once you try it for yourself you will no doubt be able to add a host of unexpected benefits.

- General and specific relaxation of muscles, providing immediate relief.

- Fibrous adhesions (knots and nodules) can be broken down.

- Dispersal of toxins from tense, knotted muscles.

- Relief from chronic neck and shoulder stiffness.

- Loosening of the scalp.

- Relaxation of the whole person.

- Increased oxygen uptake in tissues.

- Improved circulation of blood in previously congested muscles, providing extra oxygen for the brain.

- Stimulation and improvement of the circulation of the lymphatic system.

- Relief from stiffness in the neck and shoulder area.

- Restoration of joint movement in the neck and shoulders.

- Promotion of hair growth.

- Help in the relief of eyestrain and tension headaches.

- Excellent for disturbed sleep and insomnia.

- Help with mental tiredness and edginess.

- Improved concentration.

- Relief from mental and emotional stress.

# INDIAN CHAMPISSAGE

This advanced form of Indian head massage includes massage of the face, the temporo-mandibular joints (tmj), the ears and subtle energy massage (energy balancing). The added benefits of this advanced massage are both physical and mental.

## Physical Benefits

Significant improvement is noticed in the following conditions:

- Tinitus
- Temporo-mandibular joint tension (TMJ syndrome), often caused by grinding or clenching the teeth
- Sinusitis
- Migraine
- Nightmares
- Insomnia and disturbed sleep

Tinitus causes a continuous ringing or buzzing in the ears and can be a very distressing condition. Ear massage can help reduce the symptoms in less severe cases. Sinusitis is the inflammation of the sinuses in the face. This can be very painful and may make breathing difficult. The massage techniques on the face help to relieve this condition. Temporo-mandibular joint tension is also known as TMJ syndrome. It affects the muscles involved in chewing food. These muscles must exert a surprising amount of force to keep the jaw closed. This means the jaw rarely relaxes and this contributes to the overall tension in the face. TMJ syndome causes tenderness of these muscles, and this can lead to hearing and visual problems as well as headaches.

## Mental Benefits

Indian Champissage promotes:

- A sense of calmness, peace and tranquillity
- A release of anxiety
- Relief from depression
- High levels of concentration
- Clearer thinking
- Sound sleep
- The release of stagnant energy
- Chakra balancing and energetic healing

Anxiety, depression, frustration and other negative emotions have a huge bearing on our physical body, and particularly so on the face. A great many small muscles are concentrated here and they work together to produce our facial expressions, which reflect our inner thoughts and feelings.

We frequently find that the feelings we express in our daily lives are limited and often negative – joy and excitement are rarer than anxiety, fear and anger. In order to express a wider range of emotions, we must endeavour to relearn ways of moving the face. Tense jaw muscles are indicative of unexpressed anger and resentment, and releasing the tension will help release these feelings, enabling the person to let them go and move on with their lives. Champissage releases locked emotions and negative energy, making room for positive feelings. Long-term attitudes are encouraged to shift and life becomes more joyful. Over time, Champissage will soothe and heal the soul.

# WORDS OF CAUTION

Massage is one of the safest forms of therapy known to man. However, there are certain circumstances when massage should be avoided. These include when the person:

- is drunk
- is suffering from food poisoning
- is ill or has a high temperature/fever
- has had any recent accidents, injuries or surgery e.g., whiplash, head injury, concussion etc.
- is suffering from any acute infectious diseases: typhoid, diphtheria, etc.
- is undergoing medical treatment for cancer or any other serious medical condition
- is suffering from very high or very low blood pressure
- is suffering from any localized infectious/contagious skin disorders on the areas to be worked on
- is suffering from any severe inflammations
- is suffering from aneurosa – localized dilation of the blood vessels (commonly the artery in the temple/forehead area in the elderly)

If you are not a trained therapist, do **not** give Indian head massage if your partner or friend is suffering from any of the following conditions. A professional therapist or Indian head massage expert will know how to help them best.

- Osteoporosis
- Frailty
- Chronic fatigue
- Epilepsy

- Spondylitis or spondylosis in the neck
- Painful cysts
- Psoriasis

# EPILOGUE: INDIAN HEAD MASSAGE AND THE FUTURE

In this book I have tried to provide the background information and a guide to the basic techniques of a wonderful therapy, new to the West. Try it out on your friends and relatives, lovers and children. But first, why not treat yourself to a professional head massage? Only when you have experienced Indian head massage yourself will you understand its benefits and the great gift you can now give to others. I am sure many of you will have experienced body massage, however, once you have had Indian head massage you will find it becomes an inseparable part of your life. Once you learn this therapy it will be at the ends of your fingertips for a lifetime.

In founding the London Centre of Indian Champissage my aim was to make this therapy available to everyone by training others throughout the country and abroad so that every town would have a practising therapist. If you wish to know the nearest therapist to you, please do contact us and we will be happy to send you details.

My greatest hope is that there will be more research carried out into the effects of Indian head massage. As modern science develops 'cures' for more illnesses, our stressful modern life seems to be replacing them with newer, more complicated disorders. Head massage really can help. My vision of the future is this: that this massage will be available everywhere: at home, in the office, at the airport, on the plane, even in the park, and that it will become an intrinsic part of everyone's daily routine. More people giving and receiving this therapy would mean dramatic improvements in relationships. People would become calmer, happier and more loving. Make Indian head massage part of your routine and you will find an exciting transformation in the quality of your life.

# GLOSSARY

**acidosis**: an excessive production of acid in the body or an abnormal reduction of alkalinity in the blood.

**adrenaline**: this is a hormone that is produced by the adrenal glands which are situated at the top of the kidneys. When adrenaline production is increased, the blood pressure rises, the heart beat increases, along with the amount of sugar in the blood, and the stomach is immobilized, resulting in suppression of hunger.

**alopecia**: general or partial baldness which can affect both men and women.

**Ayurveda**: an Indian system of preventative medicine and health care dating back 5,000 years. Its meaning comes from two Sanskrit words: 'ayus' meaning life and 'veda' meaning 'knowledge' or 'science'. Ayurveda literally means 'the science of life'.

**carrier oil or base oil**: these are oils that are mixed with small quantities of essential oils for massage. Essential oils are extremely concentrated and should never be applied to the skin on their own. Almond oil is one of the most popular carrier oils in this country.

**cervical spondylosis**: a degenerative change in the intervertebral discs producing pain and stiffness in the neck, spreading to the shoulders and arms.

**cervical spondylitis**: inflammation of the vertebrae of the spine, creating stiffness in the spine.

**Chakra**: the literal meaning of chakra is wheel or vortex. This term is used to describe the body's energy centres. There are seven principal chakras. They are believed to exist in the etheric layer of the aura.

**ciliary muscles**: these muscles control the ability of the lens of the eye to see things at a distance and close to.

**Crohn's disease**: an inflammation of a part of the intestine, the ileum.

**dandruff**: excessive shedding of dead skin from the scalp. Dandruff can be due to dry skin or it can be caused by a fungal infection.

**diverticulum (diverticula)**: a sac or pouch formed by herniation of the wall of the intestine.

**diverticulosis**: an inflammation of the diverticula in the large intestine.

**eczema**: a skin condition where the skin becomes dry, inflamed and flaky. In advanced cases the surface of the skin breaks down and weeps fluid.

**energy centre**: see *Chakra*, *above*.

**epilepsy**: a chronic disorder characterized by sudden loss of consciousness and convulsions.

**essential oils**: these are concentrated essences, extracted from certain varieties of trees, shrubs, herbs, grasses and flowers. The therapeutic properties of essential oils have been known about and used to treat a whole spectrum of ailments throughout the world for centuries.

**extra-ocular muscles**: the muscles that help to move the eye around in its socket.

**fibrositis**: inflammatory or degenerative changes in the fibres of the muscles.

**fibrous adhesions**: this is when fibrous tissue, which should generally be separate and freely moveable, sticks together due to chronic or acute inflammation, forming knots and nodules in the muscles.

**friction**: used in Indian head massage, this technique uses light or deep pressure, and causes the skin and muscle to move over the bones of the scalp.

**hair follicles**: deep pits which extend down through the entire thickness of the skin, to the basale layer from which hair grows.

**hair root**: this is set deep in the skin. The root of the hair ends in a knob and is set upon a fibrous papilla, from which the hair appears to derive its principal nutrients. The root is the growing part of the hair which pushes the older part out.

**Indian Champissage**: an advanced form of Indian head massage which includes massage of the face, the temporo-mandibular joints, the ears and subtle massage, or energy balancing. Indian Champissage benefits the recipient on a mental, physical, spiritual and emotional level.

**irritable bowl syndrome or irritable colon (spastic colon)**: a chronic condition which causes recurring abdominal pain. It tends to occur in nervous people when under stress and strain.

**meditation**: a technique which helps the human mind to reach a state of profound stillness while remaining awake.

**osteoporosis**: an increased porousness of the bones due to lack of calcium. It is most common in women after the age of 45.

**occipital area**: the area at the base of the skull.

**psoriasis**: a non-infectious skin condition that causes the skin to become inflamed and dry, leading to flaking and scaly patches.

**rubbing**: in Indian head massage, this is a light rubbing massage technique over the surface of the skin.

**sinusitis**: a painful inflammation or blockage of the sinuses in the face.

**tinitus**: a constant ringing or high pitched sound in the ear that has no external cause.

**torticollis**: a condition that results in muscle contraction in the neck, leaving the neck bent on one side.

**toxins**: poisons produced by the overuse of the muscles.

# INDEX

'Indian head massage under the expert hands of Narendra Mehta is an experience not to be missed.' The entertainer

'Mr Narendra Mehta [is the] guru of the British Indian head massage movement. When I visited Mehta, it was the end of a long, hot, sticky day's work at the office. I felt frazzled but after half an hour of soothing Champissage I felt fresh, invigorated, yet relaxed.' Your Healthcare

'The first session [with Narendra Mehta] was unbelievable. I could feel all the tension melt away from my neck and shoulders.' Health and Fitness

'Mr Narendra Mehta is Britain's Champissage guru ...' The Express

'Regular head massage ... is guaranteed to lift you out of the hustle and bustle. This therapeutic technique, the brainchild of Narendra Mehta ... is an invaluable treatment for stress-linked troubles.' Harpers and Queen

'Mehta's style of massage dispels tension resulting in an improvement in stress-related conditions ... It is unbelievably relaxing and leaves you with a great feeling of well-being.'
Girl About Town

'Narendra Mehta has developed a scalp and head massage which combines traditional Indian techniques with his own methods. He works on the body's energy centres, the chakras, to rebalance the body's energy, so helping to promote physical and psychological well-being.' Elle